Dr Ali's
Weight
Loss
Plan

Other books by the same author:

The Integrated Health Bible

Dr Ali's Ultimate Back Book

Therapeutic Yoga

Dr Ali's Nutrition Bible

Dr Ali's
Weight
Loss
Plan

Dr Mosaraf Ali

Vermilion
LONDON

First published in Great Britain in 2005

1 3 5 7 9 10 8 6 4 2

Text copyright © Dr Mosaraf Ali, 2005
Illustrations copyright © Sarah Jarrett, 2003
Design copyright © Vermilion, 2005

Published by Ebury Publishing,
Random House, 20 Vauxhall Bridge Road, London SW1V 2SA

Random House Australia (Pty) Limited
20 Alfred Street, Milsons Point, Sydney, New South Wales 2061, Australia

Random House New Zealand Limited
18 Poland Road, Glenfield, Auckland 10, New Zealand

Random House South Africa (Pty) Limited
Enulini, 5A Jubilee Road, Parktown 2193, South Africa

The Random House Group Limited Reg. No. 954009

www.randomhouse.co.uk

A CIP catalogue for this book is available from the British Library

ISBN 0 091 90244 4

Illustrator Sarah Jarrett
Designer Jonathan Baker at seagulls
Editor Caroline Ball
Copy Editor Margaret Gilbey
Proofreader Claire Wedderburn-Maxwell
Consultant Nutritionist Fiona Hunter

With thanks to Sam Lambley, holistic massage therapist, sam_lambley@yahoo.co.uk

The chart on page 87 appears by kind permission of McGraw Hill, and is taken from
E. Braunwald's *Harrison's Principles of Internal Medicine*, Figure 75.1, p.455.

Printed and bound in Great Britain by Mackays of Chatham plc.

Contents

To David Tang, on his fiftieth

Introduction

Obesity (defined as being 20 per cent or more over the recommended weight range for your height and gender) may be a very personal problem but it is one that has become a major concern for society as a whole. Anyone involved in preventative medicine will probably rate obesity as the number one culprit behind many diseases and debilitating conditions, including heart disease and diabetes. And yet still the numbers rise. This is a health and financial time bomb ready to go off.

It is one thing to quote scary figures and say: 'Something must be done.' It is quite another to know where, at an individual level, to start. We are exhorted to eat healthily, exercise more, look after our bodies – and simultaneously we are bombarded with advertising and marketing ploys that encourage us to eat more, more often and the wrong things. Contradictory messages from the food industry and health professionals add to the fog, and from it has emerged today's fast-growing 'diet industry'. I hope my contribution towards this issue will bring about awareness of easier, safer and more effective ways of losing that extra weight.

WEIGHTY FIGURES

🍎 Adult obesity in Britain has trebled in the past twenty years; nearly two-thirds of men and over half of women are overweight or obese.

🍎 An estimated 30,000 deaths a year are linked to obesity.

🍎 It is calculated that obesity shortens life by an average of nine years.

🍎 Treating obesity and related conditions costs the NHS an estimated £500 million every year and the financial impact on the economy as a whole is as much as £2 billion.*

* All these figures come from *Tackling Obesity in England*, a report by the Comptroller and Auditor General for the National Audit office, dated 15 February 2001.

Any number of heavily marketed diets offer salvation from obesity; some even work for some people. But common to most is that they treat the symptom, i.e. excess weight, and not the person. I have always had as my starting point the advice of Hippocrates: treat the diseased not the disease. By focusing on the whole person, body and mind, rather than simply on the fat, the real problems are addressed, you can develop a sensible and healthy approach to life, and your weight adjusts to a healthy level – and stays that way.

There is not one single cure-all for excess weight because there is not one single cause. While overeating is still the most common reason for being overweight, genes play a major role in the development of obesity, as does the hypothalamus. This very important part of the brain is the control centre for the sympathetic and parasympathetic nervous systems and houses the appetite-controlling centre. Malfunction can lead to food cravings and a sluggish metabolic rate, both conditions that open the path to obesity. Body fat is also affected by gender, degree of physical activity, age and the use of certain drugs.

My observations and experience in helping patients concerned about weight gain has helped me to classify the causes of being over-weight or obese into four main categories:

- eating too much and/or exercising too little
- hormonal
- genetics and familial influences
- psychological reasons.

Some of you may recognize 'your' category instantly, but for many, weight problems will stem from a mixture of several or all of these, or may have a quite different cause from what you always supposed. This is why it is so important to understand the reasons for your being over-weight before you rush into Diet A or Exercise Regime B. There is nothing more demoralizing than working hard at something only to discover that from the outset it had no hope of success.

In the first part of this book I look in detail at how and why fat accumulates, the different types of weight gain and the causes – some unexpected as well as the usual suspects. This is followed by some detailed questions to help you assess your personal weight problems, so that you will then be able to choose the right plan – incorporating fasting, relaxation techniques, massage and exercise as well as diet – to lose weight successfully and permanently.

learning from the masters

What has enabled me to develop this successful approach to weight loss is a commitment to integrated medicine, blending the traditional, the conventional and the experimental to benefit from the best of each.

When I was a medical student in the 1970s and early 1980s in Moscow, the Soviet Health Minister was highly concerned about obesity in the population, since the state had to bear the cost of their health care. Professor Yuri Nikolaev, an eminent scientist and naturopath, campaigned to open a fasting therapy department for ailments related to diet and obesity. (He had successfully used fasting therapy to treat mental disorders at a time when electro-convulsive therapy and drugs were the most usual methods.) I was at the time doing post-graduate studies in acupuncture, but as a young enthusiast of non-conventional medicine, I began to observe everything that went on in the department and spent weekends at Professor Nikolaev's house listening to him talk about medicine and spirituality.

It was obvious that some people, particularly women, lost weight with fasting more easily than others. Professor Nikolaev noted that those who had hormonal imbalances put on fat that enzymes in the body could not breakdown so easily. That was my introduction to the idea that some types of people do not lose their excess fat as efficiently as others. Over the years I kept that in mind and researched into ways to help those whose fat was tenacious even under fasting conditions.

I returned to India to continue my training under eminent physicians of Ayurveda and Unani. Although obesity was not a major issue in India in those days, it was certainly a problem for some. I read old books on medicine by court physicians and well-known traditional medical practitioners. Few had written about obesity and weight gain. Focus was mainly on the treatment of diseases and weight loss was considered only as a side effect. Excess weight was usually seen as a problem of women, it seemed, and was always linked to hormonal imbalances. This recalled Professor Nikolaev's observations, and the effect of hormones on fat deposits and fluid retention is an important part of this book.

a different approach

The techniques I use on my patients have met with great and lasting success. Over the past twenty years I have helped thousands of people to lose weight, and I have learnt as I have taught. I have had all sorts of experiences: women wanting to slim down for their own or their children's wedding; husbands wanting to pay for their wives to lose weight as a Christmas gift; obese ladies demanding a programme that would enable them to lose a fixed target per week (and if I couldn't promise, they would not follow it). One man wanted to lose weight so that his horse could carry him without difficulty.

What are these techniques that are so successful? Three aspects of my weight loss plan are unique:

🍎 control of food cravings, using my special massage technique to work indirectly on the appetite centre in the brain. I believe its results prove my hypothesis that improving the blood supply to the subconscious brain has a beneficial effect on many areas of health, including weight

🍎 control of stomach acid, the main stimulant of appetite, by a variety of means

🍎 helping the pituitary gland's regulation of hormones that affect weight and fluid retention.

My methods also include:

🍎 an individual approach, not 'one formula for all'

🍎 retracting the stomach so that the volume of food that can be consumed is reduced drastically. This is achieved by reducing the desire to overeat and learning to recognize the body's signals of satisfaction, and by following a fasting programme that indirectly retracts the stomach

🍎 a massage technique that helps to physically flatten the unwanted cellulite or white fat, which responds so poorly to diet

🍎 a fat-burning or metabolism stimulation exercise programme that can be done at home, which helps even those who cannot do vigorous exercise or who can't go out to exercise.

What really makes the long-term difference are the lifestyle changes of this plan rather than just diet itself: forming good eating habits, regular massage, relaxation and exercise. These, with appetite and cravings under control, make you feel good as well as look good. All my patients who have undertaken the plan have said how people praised them for how well they looked. They have also remarked that they did not feel the 'pinch' of going on a weight loss diet, and called it 'sensible eating' and 'not a problem at all'. Many have adopted this approach as a lifelong practice, enjoying good health, well-being and a well-balanced weight. Some have developed an almost spiritual attitude to fasting once a week.

In short, I have created a weight loss plan that is controlled by the body's own innate healing power. That power rectifies everything that goes wrong within the body and the mind. If weight gain is a problem, it will put it right. I have only managed to help that self-regulation to work better by encouraging, without the use of drugs or intrusive methods, the conditions that allow it to function effectively.

My best wishes to you as you start on your weight loss venture. Losing weight is not always easy, and in some cases demands extraordinary perseverance, but if you follow my advice with determination, I am sure you will be successful.

Part One

Why Do We Gain Weight?

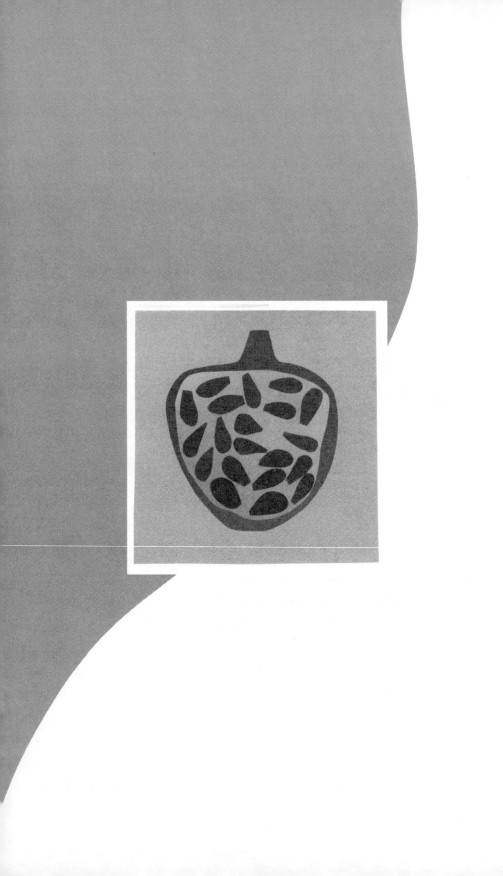

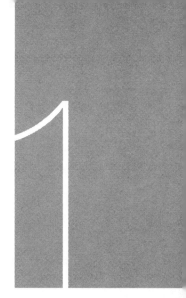

Types of Weight Gain

So far there is no perfect universal weight loss plan that works for everybody. Really, this is not surprising, as we are not all the same and so it is logical that factors such as genes, gender, metabolism, constitution and state of health and fitness should all influence how we process and store the energy we get from our food.

Having carefully observed why people put on weight and why some can and some cannot lose it, I have noted a number of important facts.

 Many people who have successfully followed a diet programme then get bored by the restrictive regime, or go on holiday and forget all about watching what they eat, and the weight all goes back on again. Most diets give you a plan to lose weight but not a plan to maintain it.

 A quite different problem faces those for whom diets have had very little effect. However little they eat, and however many different regimes they try, nothing seems to work, which makes them very frustrated and often depressed.

🍎 Some people who have never had a weight problem wake up to the fact one day that, although their diet and energy levels do not seem to have changed, they keep getting heavier.

🍎 In contrast to this, there are those for whom the opposite is true: their life undergoes a specific change – it may be giving up smoking or undergoing some traumatic event in their lives – and their weight shoots up.

Based on these and other observations and experience over the past twenty years, I have categorized weight gain into four principal causes. To lose weight on a permanent basis, you need to understand the underlying cause for your excess weight. If you have a hormonal problem then half-starving yourself will not be the answer, and if you come from generations of podgy people you may need a different approach from someone who is comfort eating to stave off emotional problems.

Type 1
eating too much, exercising too little

By far the most common cause of putting on too much weight is simply eating too much, or the wrong foods, and exercising too little. For most people, balancing what they eat and the amount of exercise they do can determine their weight. If you fall into this category you can lose weight by cutting down on what you eat, or cutting out certain foods, or exercising more. Carbohydrates and especially fats are the main source of energy in our diet: if we do not draw on this energy that our food has provided (due to a sedentary lifestyle), then storing it as fat deposits is the body's only solution.

With exercise, the demand for energy increases and the stores of fat are broken down. If you also increase the amount you eat, though, the balance will remain the same and you will not lose weight, only avoid gaining it.

There are several diets that are effective for this type of weight gain, because any regime that puts restrictions on your food intake will cause you to lose weight. In fact, the weight loss is often due to a simple change in what you eat, rather than the amount. The problem with most diets that treat this kind of weight gain is that they are not complete changes in eating habits and do not provide a workable plan for maintaining your new lower weight once you have achieved it. Cutting down on, say, sugar or fat or alcohol and doing some exercise has a beneficial effect, but once you stop and slip back into your old ways, the weight all starts piling on again.

Another common complaint about many diets is hunger pangs. It is very difficult to stick to a diet if you keep feeling hungry. In Chapter 4 I explore the many reasons our appetites are aroused and how we are encouraged to eat more than we really need.

Type 2
hormonal weight gain

The fat that commonly builds up from dietary excess or lack of exercise is called yellow fat, and it is usually deposited over the entire body. But there is another type of fat, white fat. White fat, commonly called cellulite, is accumulated as a result of hormonal changes and is found in concentrations below the navel, on the buttocks, thighs and arms, and across the breast region (in both men and women). Some hormonal imbalances, such as Cushing's syndrome, or long-term use of artificial steroids, cause fat to relocate from elsewhere on the body to the cheeks and jawline – hence the term 'moon face'.

Many of our vital functions are controlled by hormones, the levels of which are carefully balanced by the pituitary–hypothalamic area of our brain. If this gets the wrong stimuli, or is malfunctioning, the hormonal balance can be easily upset, resulting in a whole range of

FLUID RETENTION

Not all weight gain is from fat. Fluid retention, causing different parts of the body to swell, can occur for various reasons.

🍎 **Kidney problems** If the kidneys malfunction (which may be caused, for example, by an infection, cysts, stones, diabetes or lupus) their filtration system ceases to work effectively and the face, eyes and legs get 'flooded' because fluids can't get out of the system. See Chapter 5.

🍎 **Heart problems** If the heart fails to pump blood round the body efficiently it can cause fluid retention that may progressively increase. Swelling begins at the feet and ankles but in extreme cases the legs and even the abdomen become swollen, as a result of heart failure.

🍎 **Impaired circulation** Defective valves (causing varicose veins) or a blockage due to a clot (deep vein thrombosis) will impede the blood flow through the system of veins and arteries. If the blood cannot flow freely, fluid is inclined to build up in the legs.

🍎 **Malfunction in the lymphatic circulation** Just like blood, the lymph system has its own circulation, and a blockage, perhaps from infection or surgical intervention, can cause massive swelling of one or more limbs. When the legs get excessively swollen, the condition is called elephantiasis.

🍎 **Liver problems** A liver that is not functioning efficiently (see page 49) can cause a swollen abdomen that can even affect breathing (just as a woman gets easily breathless in the last stages of pregnancy).

🍎 **ADH** A hormone called ADH (antidiuretic hormone) 'instructs' the kidneys not to release water from the body if there is a danger of excess fluid loss. If a malfunction occurs this instruction may never be switched off, and water retention can be permanent. See Chapter 5.

symptoms, from cellulite deposits and fluid retention to an unregulated appetite centre.

Many women who have never had to think about their weight find that they put on weight in their late forties or as they approach the menopause. As this weight gain is primarily hormonal, it can be very difficult to shed.

The role of hormones is a complex one and so gets a chapter of its own; see Chapter 3.

Type 3
genetic and familial weight gain

Sometimes obesity runs in the family. An entire family can be fat not only because they eat the same way but also because it is in the genes. There is a particular gene (popularly referred to as the obesity gene, or ob-gene) that affects leptin, a protein produced in fat tissue. Leptin regulates how we deposit fat, so its control naturally affects our fat levels.

When scientists discovered the 'obesity gene' many thought that this was an open passport to eat and drink as they liked because they could

FOUR DIFFERENT TYPES OF PEOPLE

Hippocrates, Galen and Avicenna, the great Persian physician, divided people into four basic constitutional types: sanguine, choleric, phlegmatic and melancholic. Of these, melancholics were constitutionally underweight, cholerics often had digestive problems, so seldom became overweight, and phlegmatics were constitutionally overweight. Phlegmatics might also be described as the FFF type: fat, fair and flabby. Their skin is soft and the adipose layer is very prominent. Even sanguines, who usually 'burn up' fat successfully, find their weight gradually increasing if they are not careful.

not do anything about a genetic condition. That is not entirely true. A genetic propensity towards obesity does not, I'm afraid to say, take the responsibility out of your hands and the discovery of the obesity gene does not mean you have to be fatalistic. It is just that you have to do more and not less to control your weight.

Genes also determine our underlying body shape and weight. If both your parents are short and broad you are unlikely to be tall and willowy (even if, with an optimum diet, you may be taller than your parents). Basic body shapes run in families, just like hair and skin colour.

Weight can also be a problem that runs in the family without being strictly genetic in origin. The eating habits we learn as children become deeply ingrained, and can be passed on from one generation to another as familial, rather than truly genetic traits. Some families simply love eating. And if they share a love of food that is rich in fats and sugar, then they share the resultant weight problem too. These may be exacerbated by common habits such as spending long hours slumped in front of the TV or avoiding sport at school.

If you have a genetic disposition towards obesity, it's important not to think: I'm fat because of my genes; there's nothing I can do about it. The aim is not to emulate a very slim model or a world-class athlete, but to be a healthy weight for your height, build, sex and age – and this is certainly achievable.

Type 4
psychological reasons for weight gain

Food can be eaten for many reasons other than as fuel for the body or for pleasure. It can be a great comforter, and eating in search of an emotional uplift or for a 'sugar rush' is something that most of us indulge in from time to time, but for some people it becomes a long-term problem. Many people under stress find they eat more at these times.

Normally, the appetite centre in the hypothalamus (see Chapter 4) stimulates and suppresses appetite as it identifies low and high levels of glucose in the blood. But psychological problems can overrule these messages (which also block the hunger pangs in anorexics).

🍎 In the case of obsessive compulsive eating, all control of eating habits is lost. The appetite centre fails to stop the entire ritual attached to eating (looking at food, hand movements, chewing, swallowing), so that a sufferer can eat dozens of ice creams, empty out packs of cookies, devour a whole block of cheese within minutes, without any check from the appetite centre. The mind goes into a state where eating brings neither comfort nor satisfaction. In times of stress or anxiety, the desire to eat something is uncontrollable, however full the stomach. This ritualistic eating pattern is the same as other obsessive compulsive behavioural patterns such as constant hand-washing or pulling out hair, where the action itself provides some sort of relief. A huge increase in weight is inevitable. Since the hypothalamus is involved, its other functions are also likely to get out of kilter, resulting in increased fluid retention and hormonal problems, leading to yet more weight gain.

🍎 Binge-eating is a milder form of obsessive compulsive disorder, and also has psychological causes. As soon as bulimics feel stressed, they try to divert the mind by eating; the taste of food and the process of eating is calming and helps to overcome the stress temporarily. Of course, it does nothing to resolve the actual cause of the stress, and if this persists then bingeing can recur several times a day. Bulimia is a more severe form of this, in which sufferers force themselves to vomit after a bingeing session.

People who are affected to this degree are, of course, in the minority, but if you follow the questions in the Self-assessment chapter (see pages 78–9) you may find, as many people do, that comfort eating plays a part in your weight problems.

other contributors to weight gain

There are a number of other factors than can contribute to weight gain, such as:

Muscle bulk: Gram for gram, muscles weigh more than fat, so heavy exercise can cause your weight to increase because of the build-up of muscle bulk. Body builders and sumo wrestlers are huge in size but their weight is in their muscles. In following a vigorous weight loss programme that combines diet and exercise, initial weight loss can be rapid as it is from fluids and reduction of fat, but then it disappointingly slows down as muscles build up. This needs to be taken into account when comparing or recording weights, and is another illustration of how individual we are.

Giving up smoking: Putting on weight is a major concern for people who give up or intend to give up smoking. Why are the two connected? Smoking's 'feel-good' factor comes in part because nicotine dilates the blood vessels and allows more blood to flow through. As the appetite centre in the hypothalamus is well supplied with blood, and therefore with glucose, smoking can keep the appetite suppressed. After giving up smoking, the opposite happens and the appetite centre sends out messages of increased appetite and in particular a craving for sweet things. The metallic taste in the mouth after giving up smoking also increases the demand for something sweet.

To the many young teenage girls who take up smoking in order to stay slim, nicotine's appetite-dampening properties may seem a great idea, but they are just building up problems for the future.

Chronic Fatigue Syndrome and ME: CFS, often flippantly and misleadingly called 'yuppie flu', is frequently labelled as a psychological problem. In my opinion, CFS is a multifactorial condition, to which a viral infection, poor supply of glucose and oxygen to the brain and yeast or fungal overgrowth in the gut, can all contribute. (Epstein Barr virus triggers CFS in up to 30 per cent of cases and sufferers can continue to be affected for years from its debilitating drain on energy even though viral activity is negligible. This is the severest form of CFS, and is called myalgic encephalomyelitis or ME.) CFS often leads to a marked weight gain because it combines a craving for sugar with such low energy levels that exercise becomes impossible.

Prescription drugs: HRT drugs and steroids such as cortisone are well known for causing a rise in weight (Chapter 3 explains the reason for this), but other drugs such as antibiotics and antidepressants can also cause weight gain.

Alcohol: Alcohol contributes to weight increase in several ways. Just like an alcohol-based cleaner soaks up grease, alcohol helps fat to be absorbed effectively. Alcohol, especially white wine or champagne, before a meal enhances your appetite. It is also highly calorific and quickly absorbed, so more of the food eaten with or after the alcohol is perceived by the body as surplus to its energy requirements and so is stored as fat.

Old age: As we age we tend to graduate more towards our natural body type. While some people find they become positively skinny in old age, for many fat seems part and parcel of the ageing process. This does not have to be so. Being overweight 'just because you are old' is often unnecessary and is due to the failure to recognize that our diet needs to adapt to our ageing bodies.

Continuing to eat three full meals a day, even when your mobility is restricted, or having a diet far too concentrated on bread, butter, cheese, salt, sweets and puddings will usually account for the increase

CASE STUDY

A bulging tummy is not always due to fat. When a famous French actress was offered a role in a film, she quickly wanted to lose some weight she had put on around her middle. She came to London to see me, and as she entered my room I knew exactly what the problem was.

As she lay on the couch I asked her to place her hands on the sides of her abdomen and note the temperature. 'Warm', she said. Then I asked her to move her hands to the centre of her abdomen and she immediately noticed it was much cooler. I asked her to lift both legs about 15 cm above the couch and told her to look at her tummy. 'That's strange,' she remarked, 'it's bulging more, like an inflated balloon.'

I explained that although she had some excess fat around the hips and buttocks, her tummy was bulging because of a hernia. The sheaths of abdominal ligaments that encase the straight muscles in the front (the 'abs') are joined in the centre of the abdomen, along the thickened hairline. Excessive abdominal gas, pregnancy, lack of exercise and sometimes abdominal surgery can cause them to open up and the two edges to become loose and separate. Habitually lying on your side for a sleep immediately after heavy meals can also cause this common type of hernia. When a person stands up, the intestines form a pouch under the skin, giving the false impression of a large tummy. When lying down, the pouch disappears. Because the muscles and blood vessels no longer meet, the central area of the abdomen feels cooler than the sides.

I recommended a low-fat diet for a month and suggested she wear an elastic abdominal support. She lost the weight quickly and, when I later went to see the film, I was delighted that she looked perfect, with no bulges.

in weight. Pre-packaged, ready-to-eat meals may seem like a great convenience, but they also exacerbate indigestion, constipation, bloating and gas. Additional weight puts strain on the joints (think of all those hip and knee replacements) as well as the heart. In countries where ancient traditions are followed, such as Japan, elderly people generally eat less. They know very well that their digestive power is weaker and that eating late or at night is not good, so they develop a habit of eating some breakfast, a normal lunch and only a very light dinner. In India elderly people eat fruit or rice puddings or drink milk for dinner – never a full meal.

Even from these brief descriptions I expect you recognize some familiar scenarios; quite probably you feel you are a mixture of more than one category. The following chapters will explain in more detail what is involved in different types of weight gain, and answering the questions in the Self-assessment chapter (see Chapter 8) will also help clarify matters. You will then be ready to lose that weight for ever!

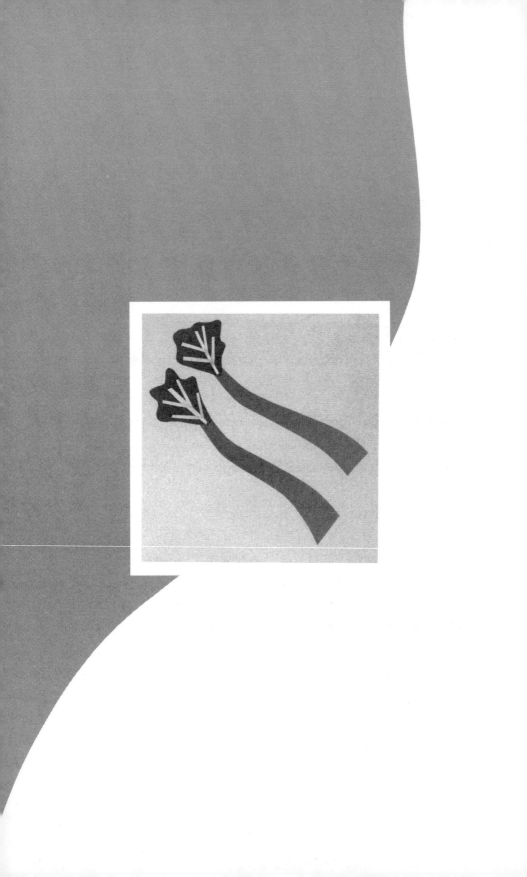

All About Fat

Fat is vital. Fat gives contours to our bodies and cushions our bottoms so that we don't have to sit uncomfortably on muscles or bones. Fat protects our heart from bumping against the lungs and the chest cavity as we jog, do a headstand or even just turn over in bed. Fat helps protect the vulnerable milk-producing glands in the breast and allows our eyeballs the freedom to swivel around as they do.

Nature uses fat in some very clever ways. Our intestines are bound by two sets of ligaments to stop them from becoming entangled, rather like spokes on a bicycle wheel. Fat deposits on the membranes located in the inner 'rims' of the intestines protect the numerous blood vessels, nerves and lymphatic vessels. These fat deposits also keep the intestines intact so that food can pass through smoothly without any obstructions. (It is excess fat deposits in these membranous sheaths that is the cause of a bulging beer belly.)

storing energy

Food enables us to function, not just giving us the energy to run or dance or the mental stamina to do a busy job, but all manner of things that go on without our ever thinking about them, from repairing and replacing cells to secreting hormones and maintaining our immune system.

All these functions are carried out by special energy-producing compounds called ATP, which are largely synthesized in the mitochondria or power stations located inside the cells of the body. Cells need energy all the time to support themselves and carry out their work. They procure energy by breaking down the three main products that form the bulk of our nourishment: carbohydrate, protein and fat.

Carbohydrates are broken down first, as this is the quickest and easiest chemical process. Carbohydrate is stored (as glycogen) in the liver and in the muscles. Both the liver and muscles need a quick source of energy to carry out their functions and nature has given them this facility to synthesize and store energy in their tissues. However, only about three per cent of the body's stored energy originates as carbohydrates, so when they run out of carbohydrates, because of short supply or increased demand for energy, they then turn to fat to release energy (protein is rarely broken down to produce energy, except *in extremis*, as

LIVING OFF OUR FAT

Those who go on arduous expeditions to the polar regions intentionally put on fat by eating fatty foods, extra protein and drinking olive oil. On the journey their energy expenditure will be several times greater than usual, and this fat will act as an energy reserve in times of extreme calorie demand. It also means they have to haul around less food. A similar process is at work in bears, who fatten themselves up during the summer months and then live off these stores of fat during their deep winter hibernation.

proteins are the structural blocks of the body itself). So, fat is the main energy reserve in the body. When broken down in the body, fats provide on average twice as much energy as carbohydrate, gram for gram.

In normal circumstances, fats account for 10–12 per cent of our body weight. When supply of fats exceeds the demand for energy, the excess is stored in fat deposits around the body. This is a dangerous thing.

fat digestion

Carbohydrates and proteins are broken down by various enzymes into glucose and amino acids, which are absorbed by the capillaries of the intestines and transported to the liver. Fats, however, cannot follow the same route, as they are formed of droplets of oil, which repel water.

Instead, bile, secreted by the liver, emulsifies these oil droplets to enable them to be absorbed by the intestine walls. From here they diffuse into the tiny lymphatic vessels and join the main lymphatic system and, ultimately, the bloodstream. So, because it is completely

THE CONSTRUCTION OF FAT

Fat (also known as adipose tissue) consists of large cells or adipocytes. Each cell is filled with a single enormous droplet of lipid or oil, so that the nucleus and other cellular structures are squeezed to one side, making the cells resemble a ring.

When food is scarce, or in old age, or during a weight loss programme, the fat cells deflate like a collapsing balloon as the lipid content in them disappears. However, these fat cells are not killed or broken down – they simply shrink, and when their fat content is replaced they swell up again. If fat cells do disappear or are destroyed – for example, if they are removed by liposuction – other cells in the area convert into fat cells and are inflated with lipids, so once again the fat reappears within a short period of time.

bypassed, the liver cannot exercise any control over the amount of fat in the bloodstream in the way that it screens proteins and carbo-hydrates. Control over the fats or lipids in our body, therefore, must come more directly from us. If our bile secretion is adequate and there are no problems with absorption through the gut walls, almost all the fat we consume is absorbed.

types of fat

When you think of body fat, you think of the bulging bits you would rather be without. But lipids (lipos just means fat) in the body are of many types, for example:

lipid type	function	where found
fatty acids	energy source	absorbed from foods or synthesized in the body
glycerides e.g. triglyceride	energy source, insulation, body contours	stored as body fat
steroids e.g. cholesterol	structural component of cells, hormones, bile	in blood

 Fatty acids are either absorbed from food or synthesized in the body. They are used in the body as a source of energy. Saturated fatty acids increase the risk of heart disease and other circulatory problems arising from plaque formation in the blood vessels. The dietary sources of saturated fatty acids are butter, fatty meat, cream, ice cream and so on. Vegetable oils, such as olive oil and corn oil, have unsaturated fatty acids. These are relatively safe for the heart and vascular system.

A special type of fatty acid called omega-3 is present in fish flesh and fish oils. For reasons that are not altogether clear, omega-3 fatty acid helps prevent heart disease, rheumatoid arthritis and osteoarthritis – Eskimos whose traditional diet is rich in omega fatty acids do not suffer from heart disease, even though they consume a lot of fat.

🍎 *Glycerides* are formed from the fatty acids in our diet, and as di-glycerides and triglycerides they serve as effective insulation (heat loss through fat is only about a third of that through other tissues), act as cushions against shocks to our vital organs and in times of need they yield the fatty acids that provide energy. Triglycerides absorb the fat-soluble vitamins (A, D, E and K), but also drugs or even toxins that arrive in the body fluids, so an accumulation has both positive and negative effects.

🍎 *Steroids* are an important and useful form of lipid. There are several types. Some, such as testosterone and oestrogen, carry out hormonal functions, while other steroids are regulators, such as adrenaline, the main stress hormone, and calcitriol, the regulator of minerals in the body. Cholesterol, also a steroid, forms part of cell membranes and is useful for cell division.

Artificial steroids, such as prednisone or hydrocortisone, are used to treat many disorders and are often considered 'life-saving drugs', but they have also become associated with unpleasant side effects, including weight gain. This is a two-edged sword, because steroids are useful to the body. For example, the bile salts that form bile, the most important compound that facilitates the digestion and absorption of lipids (the very component from which they are derived), are also steroids. Next time you hear the word 'steroids', think also of the useful ones that form the building blocks of many important compounds in the body.

Cholesterol is the main culprit in heart disease, as it clogs the arteries of the heart and other organs and reduces blood flow. Although most of the cholesterol in blood is dietary (meat, cream, egg yolk) the body also produces its own, which cannot be controlled by diet. Exercise can help to a certain degree, but cholesterol levels in the blood are difficult to control, especially if it is an inherited trait. Certain oils, such as omega-3 fish oils, help to regulate cholesterol, as do garlic and some herbs.

too much of a good thing

Fat, therefore, has many uses, and we would not survive without it. Our trouble is when it becomes an excess.

This is not a natural state of affairs. Unless they are force-fed or restricted to an unnatural lifestyle, as battery chickens are, or have a hormonal abnormality, animals grow to a certain size and remain that way, as their genes dictate. It is sad that humankind has stopped communication with nature. We no longer consider ourselves part of nature. We decide on our habits and living conditions without stopping for a moment to think about what nature wants us to do, what ancestral, cultural or religious habits have taught us about maintaining our physical and mental health. We disregard everything that is traditional.

EARLY GROWTH

Young babies gain approximately 600 g a week over the first month and 1 kg per month for the first year. Thereafter a child puts on about 2 kg in weight per year for the first 10 years. This is normal growth, and until about 10 years of age, paediatricians concern themselves with the height and the weight of a child in combination. Once puberty is reached the height is a concern only when it is too slow. Growth in height continues to around the age of 22 or 23, but growth in weight may continue unabated if we get out of sync with nature.

Too much fat is not just a matter of not fitting into stylish clothes or feeling embarrassed by bulges. Fat is also a troublemaker. It puts an extra workload on the heart, causes aches and pains as it exerts pressure on joints and discs and makes exercise, even basic movement, problematic, leading to an unhealthy vicious circle.

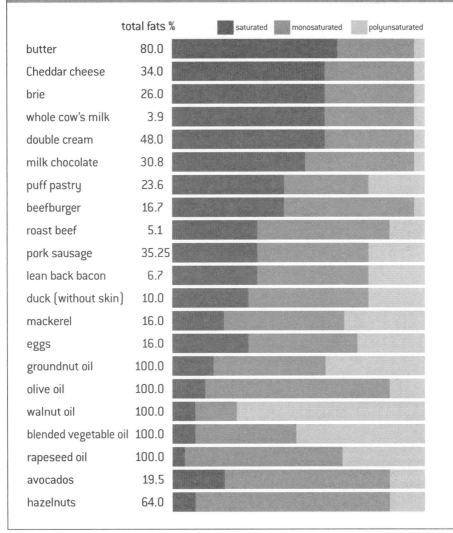

FAT CONTENT OF COMMON FOODS

	total fats %	saturated	monosaturated	polyunsaturated
butter	80.0			
Cheddar cheese	34.0			
brie	26.0			
whole cow's milk	3.9			
double cream	48.0			
milk chocolate	30.8			
puff pastry	23.6			
beefburger	16.7			
roast beef	5.1			
pork sausage	35.25			
lean back bacon	6.7			
duck (without skin)	10.0			
mackerel	16.0			
eggs	16.0			
groundnut oil	100.0			
olive oil	100.0			
walnut oil	100.0			
blended vegetable oil	100.0			
rapeseed oil	100.0			
avocados	19.5			
hazelnuts	64.0			

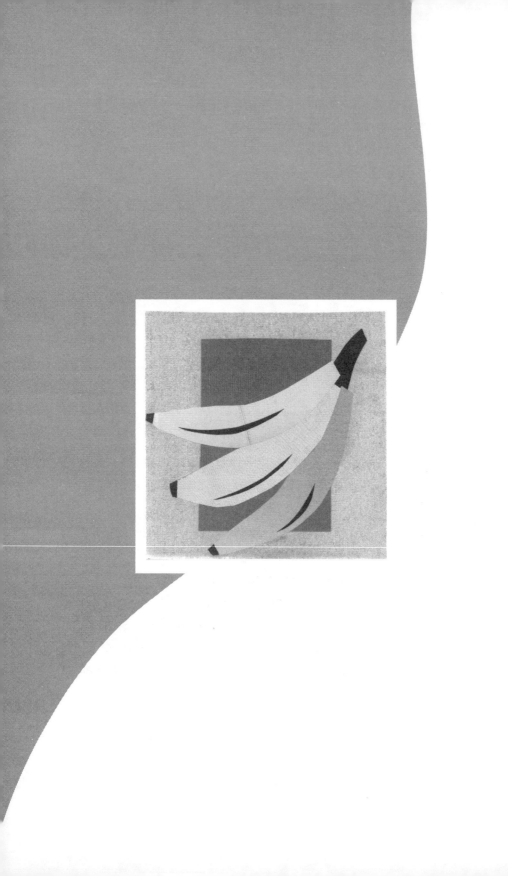

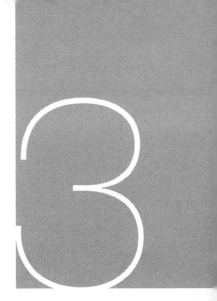

All About Hormones

An amazing range of our body's functions – reproduction, growth, metabolism, immune system, labour, sugar level in blood, blood synthesis, milk secretion, stress reactions, kidney function; in fact, most of our involuntary, subconscious functions – are controlled by hormones. Some have a profound influence on our weight control.

Keeping all our hormones properly regulated is a complex business but one, thank goodness, that our body usually manages to do perfectly, without any thought on our part. However, all sorts of things can cause an upset in the delicate balance, and some of these affect our weight, including:

🍎 wrong or mixed messages reaching the appetite centre in the brain (pituitary–hypothalamus)
🍎 a slowed metabolic rate (thyroid)

- increased fluid retention (pituitary–hypothalamus)
- excess production of oestrogen or androgens (ovaries or testes)
- medication, ranging from cortisone-based treatments to the contraceptive pill.

HOW DO HORMONES WORK?

Probably the most familiar hormones are those to do with sex: testosterone and oestrogen. But just as the body must be kept in careful balance (and an imbalance can, as you will see, affect weight as well as our 'maleness' or 'femaleness'), we have many other hormones which, when released in a particular circumstance, allow the body to respond appropriately.

A well-known example is the 'fight-or-flight' response. When a hare, for instance, sees a fox, a message of fright causes the pituitary gland to secrete a chemical that tells the adrenal glands to release adrenaline, a hormone, into the blood. This triggers a full-alert response: the heart rate goes up, muscles tense, the body temperature and metabolic rate rise and breathing is faster, all coordinated to gear the hare to face battle or to flee. (It is adrenaline, too, that drives the fox in the chase.)

This ability for one stimulus to cause a wide range of reactions is an efficient way of functioning, and quite unlike a simple nerve reaction such as the knee-jerk response, when stimulating one nerve (by sharply tapping the tendon below the kneecap) causes one response (the jerk). Moreover, when the stimulus on a nerve stops, the response stops, whereas with hormones the reaction continues for longer. The relevance for weight of this important difference is that a particular hormonal condition has a continuing or prolonged effect on the body – even an instant change (such as coming off a particular medication) will not show results straight away.

the pituitary, the hypothalamus and hormone regulation

The pituitary gland might be called the master controller of all hormones. Hormones are not automatically secreted every time a situation arises. The brain analyses an external stimulus and sends a message to the hypothalamus, which is the 'headquarters' of the autonomous or involuntary nervous system. The hypothalamus in turn sends a message to the pituitary, which secretes hormone factors that stimulate the relevant glands to release hormones into the blood. So all hormones are directly or indirectly controlled by the pituitary–hypothalamus area of the brain, which ensures quantity and quality of the highest order.

The hypothalamus houses the centre that controls hunger and appetite, the digestive process and fluid retention. These are obviously important in relation to weight, and malfunctioning of the hypothalamus can be at the root of food cravings, fluid retention and poor digestion, all of which lead to weight problems. These affect weight directly, but the hormones secreted by the glands that the pituitary stimulates can also have a noticeable effect on weight.

The thyroid: The thyroid curves across the windpipe in front of the neck – this is the gland that, when malfunctioning, can swell up to produce a goitre. Thyroid hormones (the main one is thyroxine) affect every cell in the body; in growing children, for instance, they are essential for developing bones, muscles and nerves.

If your thyroid's hormone production is high, your metabolic rate rises, enhancing the rate at which you burn glucose to produce heat and energy. A very high metabolic rate means an over-fast heart rate, increased sweating, muscle tension, diarrhoea and, because stores of energy are being burnt so fast, weight loss.

When thyroid hormone production is low, the effect is the opposite: a very slow metabolic rate leads to swellings under the skin, hair loss, dry skin, low body temperature, poor periods in women, chronic fatigue, muscle weakness – and formation of fat deposits and water retention.

🍎 *Adrenal glands:* The adrenal glands are located above the kidneys. They produce different steroid hormones collectively known as corticosteroids. These are vital to our survival and also influence our weight. Aldosterone controls water and mineral balance by acting on the kidneys, and over-production of this hormone may cause water retention and increased blood pressure. Over-production of glucocorticoids leads to an increased appetite and redistribution of fat in the body, including to the face.

Synthetic forms of glucocorticoids, hydrocortisone or cortisone, are used to treat allergies, auto-immune disease, inflammation and as an overall booster to fight various ailments. Their side effects, including weight gain in the same pattern as natural over-production, can be alarming. Taking synthetic glucocorticoids also suppresses the body's own production, as the body misinterprets the synthetic version as its own, and reduces its output.

Cortisol is the stress hormone. It triggers a release of glucose for instant energy and stimulates the appetite to supply additional energy, ready for 'fight or flight'. However, fighting or fleeing is not usually the answer to the sort of stresses we face these days, and so these extra energy reserves are not usually used up. Instead they are stored as fat, deposited on the face or tummy. This is why prolonged or repeated stress, causing regular over-production of cortisol, can lead to an increase in weight.

The adrenal glands also secrete a small amount of androgen, which has repercussions for both men and women (see below).

🍎 *Insulin:* The pancreas secretes enzymes that facilitate digestion and a hormone, insulin, to metabolize glucose. When blood sugar rises above a certain level, the brain gets alarmed as the sugar may clog up smaller blood vessels. It signals to the pancreas to secrete insulin, which quickly removes excess glucose from the blood by aiding absorption of glucose by cells and by converting glucose to glycogen (a form of starch) for storage in the liver and muscles.

Insulin is instrumental in weight increase because it helps fat cells absorb fatty acids from the blood. Fat cells also absorb the excess glucose from the blood and convert it into lipids. This way the fat cells get inflated with lipids and this results in fat formation and weight gain.

* *Androgens and oestrogen:* If the pituitary over-stimulates the adrenal cortex, then along with other hormones, androgens or male hormones are also secreted, both in men and women. In women this may cause facial and body hair growth, deposits of fat around the abdomen and muscular development. Since the female body naturally reacts against changes like this, its response is to convert or 'aromatize' the excess male hormones into an oestrogen-like hormone, oesterone. This is deposited in white fat or cellulite, typically on the thighs, buttocks, breasts, arms and waist.

GYNAECOMASTIA

Overweight men often acquire fatty deposits across the chest, giving the appearance of breasts, but there is a quite different condition, not related to obesity, called gynaecomastia. Over-stimulation of a man's adrenal glands sometimes produces oestrogen instead of androgen, or the ratio between testosterone and oestrogen may become unbalanced. This can cause the mammary glands to develop, resulting in actual breasts. Many men affected in this way are very self-conscious of having large breasts and they hate to swim or do anything that means exposing their body.

Men whose weight gain is primarily hormonal also develop a feminine distribution of white fat or cellulite below the belly button and on the arms and thighs. Men and women who are obese due to hormonal malfunctions often resemble each other, the men becoming more feminized and women more masculine.

Just as a fever or an allergic reaction is an unwelcome but healthy sign of the body actively fighting an unwanted 'invader', deposits of cellulite fat

POLYCYSTIC OVARY DISEASE

This is a classic example of how obesity and hormone disturbances are related. In this case the pituitary is confused by excess androgen production in the ovaries and adrenal glands. As androgens are aromatized, deposits of cellulite increase, but continued excess androgen production leads to infertility, hirsutism (male-pattern hair growth) and amenorrhoea (lack of periods or irregular menstrual cycle).

The pituitary also secretes two major hormones that control the functions of the ovaries: follicle stimulating hormone (FSH) and luteinizing hormone (LH). If a pituitary is not responding correctly and continues to secrete LH in excess it will cause the ovaries to synthesize more androgens. In polycystic ovary disease (PCOD), the FSH level from the pituitary drops, causing a reduction in the conversion of androgens to the main ovarian oestrogen. We have seen that, because the female body does not want to become masculinized, excess androgens are aromatized as oesterone and stored as cellulite. So the result of increased LH and decreased FSH secretion by a malfunctioning pituitary is more and more of that hard-to-move white fat.

Sadly, gynaecologists who treat PCOD, or infertility caused by it, insist that patients lose weight first. These women struggle very hard and hope that losing weight may cure their problem. In my opinion the weight problem is a result of the hormonal imbalance primarily caused by pituitary malfunction, and it is restoring this balance that will resolve both problems.

could be said to be a healthy sign that the body has dealt with unwanted hormones. But nobody wants the unattractive, pitted look of cellulite.

Because cellulite deposits are not directly related to excessive eating or poor exercise – think of them as a hormone factory outside the ovaries or adrenal glands – these stores of fat do not respond to diet or exercise very well. For the most effective treatment, see Chapter 14.

menopause

Many women have noticed that, with the onset of the menopause, they have put on weight and can find no explanation for it if they eat and exercise just the same as they used to. The answer is, unsurprisingly, hormonal. As a woman's reproductive function comes to an end, the secretion of oestrogen naturally reduces. The effect of this is to change the balance between oestrogen and androgens, the male hormones. To restore harmony, the body's reaction may be to aromatize what it perceives as excess androgens – resulting in more cellulite deposits. Fluid retention may also increase at this time, and as the menopause can be a stressful time, it may trigger psychological responses such as food cravings or comfort eating.

hysterectomy

The surgical removal of the uterus, and sometimes also the ovaries, may be necessary for a number of reasons, including a prolapsed uterus, fibroids or cancer. Removing the uterus, especially if the ovaries are active, brings about hormonal changes. This leads to weight gain following the hormonal pattern. A course of HRT after removal of the ovaries can also bring about a rapid increase in weight. Problems may also be exacerbated while psychological adjustments are faced, and binge-eating is not an uncommon side effect.

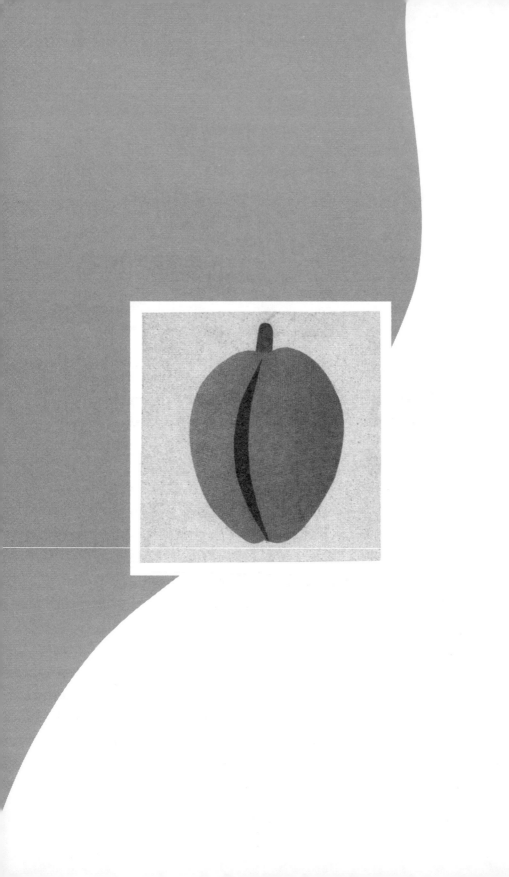

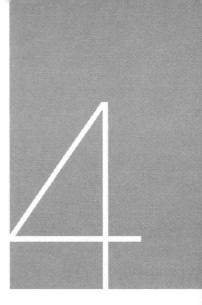

Why Do We Eat Too Much?

Our appetite for food varies enormously, from person to person, from day to day and from mood to mood. It can be depleted by complaints such as fever, diarrhoea or depression, enhanced by physical exercise, low blood pressure or convivial company, and can be distorted by a number of psychological problems. In ordinary health and ordinary conditions, one of the main triggers that urges us to eat is the appetite centre in our brain.

signals from the appetite centre

The main appetite centre is located in the hypothalamus. It is stimulated by several factors but the principal one is the level of glucose reaching it through blood or the cerebrospinal fluid that provides the brain with nutrients (principally glucose, oxygen and minerals).

An empty stomach and a build-up of acid in the stomach send a message to the conscious brain to create a sense of hunger. Acting on this, the appetite centre produces a range of psychological and physical drives to eat: increased saliva production, an anticipatory churning

BYPASSING THE TASTEBUDS

As well as providing our sense of taste, with which we associate so much of the pleasure of food, the tastebuds on our tongue send out other signals. They tell the stomach about the sort of food it can expect and they forewarn the appetite centre that the body's need for food is being fulfilled. Tastebuds therefore play a big role in controlling appetite.

Imagine a meal mostly of meat and rice cooked in ghee, for example, or a roast joint with potatoes. Digesting a meal like this requires a lot of energy and effort, so the tastebuds will soon signal the hypothalamus to stop the stimulus to eat. Eaten slowly and savoured, allowing the tastebuds to do their job, a message of satisfaction will reach the appetite centre fairly quickly, before the stomach is full.

If you eat too quickly the tastebuds do not get the chance to do this sort of evaluation in time, and the feeling of satisfaction arrives too late, when receptors in the stomach walls are registering signs of fullness. By then, large amounts of food have been consumed. Chewing and tasting food properly can affect your level of appetite and help to regulate the volume of food you consume.

Eating too fast also means you swallow a lot of air, which distends the stomach. Given this treatment regularly, the stomach walls get stretched with each meal, lose their elasticity and become flaccid. Larger amounts of food have to be eaten before the receptors can feel the sensation of fullness. The volume of the stomach is forcibly increased by the silly habit of eating fast. The result is obvious: those who eat a lot will always feel the need to eat a lot, irrespective of what their body requires.

in the stomach and a heightened awareness of the need for food, which begins the process of finding, preparing and eating it. We are all familiar with these. It is said that 'a hungry man is an angry man' because when these messages are ignored or cannot be satisfied they can cause anger, frustration, anxiety and great irritability – all this just because the body has been told it needs food.

Once our stomach is full or the circulating glucose level in the blood commands the appetite centre to stop the drive to eat, we feel satisfied and our desire to eat leaves us.

This is all as it should be. And if we always listened to our bodies, and our hypothalamus was in good working order, then we would only eat what we needed, when we needed it. Our appetite, however, can be easily over-stimulated or the messages that we have eaten enough can be ignored or over-ridden. How does this happen?

The enticement to eat more than we need comes from two types of sources: outside influences, such as tempting advertising and food displays, and messages from within our own bodies, and the interplay between them.

cravings

There is a saying: 'Sensible people eat for their stomach and fools eat for their eyes and taste.' Eating good food should be an enjoyable experience, but some people see or smell food and they go crazy. Coffee shops play on these inner cravings: they know the smell of coffee is irresistible and they attract people like bees to flowers. In addition, certain types of food become associated with positive emotions and something like alcohol or chocolate can become a prop to produce a similar sense of contentment that others might get from music or sport.

The most common cravings are for simple carbohydrates (sugar, sweets, ice cream), as these bring the quickest reaction. It is well known that something sweet – a bar of chocolate or a glucose tablet – will bring fast relief to hunger pangs. In fact, this happens even before digestion has begun. As soon as the tastebuds in the tongue receive signals of something sweet, they send a message, via the conscious brain and the hypothalamus, that the liver can release some of its stored glycogen as more will be on the way. Released as glucose into the blood, this quickly reaches the appetite centre, satisfying its demand for glucose, and the cravings go away ... for a short while.

Not all cravings are for sweet things. They can also be for savoury, especially salty, flavours such as crisps and nuts, and for fiery tastes. Chillies are well known for their addictive nature. Chillies make you flush, sweat and give you a heady feeling; as the heart rate goes up and pumps more blood you receive a spurt of energy. It is like taking a drug (those who chew tobacco experience a similar effect). You want to repeat the experience, and the more hot chillies you eat the more you want to eat, and the hotter you want them. In hot climates, chillies are used to spark flagging appetites, but the proliferation of Mexican, South Asian and Far Eastern restaurants has radically changed many people's eating habits in more temperate zones, contributing to weight problems.

THE CHILLI HABIT

Many curry dishes are high in ghee or oil and salt, and chilli dishes often come with cheese. Both are usually accompanied by quantities of carbohydrates in the form of rice or flat breads. When they are consumed regularly – particularly with copious amounts of beer and followed by sweets or ice cream 'to put out the fire' – they quickly become part of a diet that makes you put on weight. But the addictive nature of the fiery spices makes them hard to give up ...

stomach acid

Acidity is an appetite stimulator. An empty stomach is inclined to be acid, which is why acidity in the stomach, even if it is not empty, makes us want to eat. A number of things cause stomach acidity to increase:

🍎 **acidic food:** as well as vinegary foods and citrus fruits this includes sour apples and grapes and other fruit such as pineapples, kiwi fruit and berry fruits

🍎 **food that is very spicy or very hot (in temperature):** anything that irritates the delicate lining of the gut is likely to cause hypersecretion of acid

🍎 **hot, strong tea:** the combination of a very hot liquid and the tannin in tea irritates the stomach lining and increases acidity

🍎 **not chewing rough or hard food thoroughly:** when the stomach has to do the job of the teeth in grinding food, the gastric juices become very acidic

🍎 **irregular meals:** skipping meals leaves an empty stomach, which becomes acidic

🍎 **alcohol:** except for alkaline drinks such as Campari and bitters, alcohol can cause acidity problems on an empty stomach

🍎 **nicotine:** smoking regularly or chewing tobacco can cause acidity, as nicotine causes mucus discharge in the stomach

🍎 **medicines:** some medicinal drugs such as steroids and painkillers as well as high-dose vitamin C supplements (over 1000 mg)

🍎 **stress:** a body tensed by stress needs more energy, triggering acid secretion to increase appetite

🍎 **Helicobacter pylori:** this bacterium thrives in the gut wall, causing inflammation. The stomach then secretes more acid, which can lead to gastritis and ulcers.

THE CREAM TEA DIET

Since sweet and fatty foods appease the desire for food almost immediately, a diet of cream teas may seem to be the perfect answer! Certainly, the fats (cream and butter) and carbohydrates (sugar, jam and scones) will quickly satisfy the appetite centre – and probably the pleasure centre – but sadly the news is not all good.

The quick supply of glucose that sweet foods provide is very soon used up, resulting in just as quick a drop in glucose levels – creating an even greater demand for more.

Fatty or oily food suppresses hunger pangs for a while, but also encourages the production of more acid in the stomach to wash away the fats. Once the oil or fat lining the stomach is washed away it leaves an excess of acid. (This is what can cause indigestion and heartburn after a fatty or oily meal.) And excess acidity stimulates the appetite.

Sweet and fatty foods are very high in energy. This means that they supply much more than you will be able to use up, and so a great deal of what you consume will turn into fat deposits.

The traditional order in which the courses of a meal are eaten reflects the effect of acidic and sweet foods on our appetite. Starting with a sweet, creamy dessert would completely ruin your appetite for what follows, whereas alcohol (especially white wine and sparkling wine), nuts, crisps and orange juice stimulate the appetite. In the Middle East, Russia and other places salads are served before a main meal, as the enzymes in the raw food sharpen the appetite.

When I was a medical student we were taught about a condition called anhydric gastritis or inflammation of a stomach low in acid. It was considered to be bad because patients became anaemic and had a tendency to tumours. Nowadays, it is rare to diagnose someone with low stomach acidity. Changing eating habits and a faster pace of life have put pressure on our bodies: more stress = more demand for energy = more demand for food = more acid = more eating.

This chain culminates in our overeating, especially if we do not listen to the signals our bodies give us.

Regulation of stomach acid is thus a key element of my weight loss plans. Not only does it control the appetite, but it also improves digestion. Most symptoms of bad digestion – irritable bowel syndrome (IBS), indigestion, gas, cramps, burping, etc. – can also be linked to excess stomach acid.

APPETITE STIMULANTS

- citrus fruits, pineapple
- pickles
- chilli, ginger, garlic and spices; also some herbs (especially thyme)
- cheese
- white wine, champagne, brandy
- enticing colour, attractive presentation
- smell of coffee and chocolate.

a 'starved' hypothalamus

Anything that causes the appetite centre in the hypothalamus to receive less than the optimum amount of glucose will trigger it to send out signals for more – in other words, to make you feel that you need to eat.

Unless you really are starving, reduced levels of glucose reaching the hypothalamus are likely to be due to a restriction or distortion of the arteries that feed this area of the brain. For how this comes about, and how it can be alleviated, see Chapter 6.

office life

The pace of working life is very fast nowadays. Computerization was intended to make life easier, but in fact workloads have increased. Food is delivered to your desk so you do not even have to leave it for lunch. You work and eat at the same time, swallowing food without paying it proper attention. Sitting in front of a computer makes your neck tighten up. If this interferes with the hypothalamus's supply of glucose, it will make you crave snacks such as chocolate, crisps and sugary drinks. Long hours and a tiring job leave little energy for physical exercise. All these things – a sedentary life, stress, poor posture, snacking and grazing rather than regular mealtimes – will naturally lead to putting on weight.

Wining and dining clients or colleagues may be aimed at making business run more smoothly, but business lunches and dinners do not help your digestion or weight control at all. Food and drinks are generally chosen to please the palate and the eye rather than to cater to the body's needs. If your guest orders something rich and calorific, or insists on more wine, it might be perceived as rude not to follow suit. Celebrations of success, office birthdays, 'team-building' get-togethers all too often mean repeated indulgence in food and drink that can be difficult to avoid.

socializing

Social occasions are a major factor in weight increase. If you go out for dinner, then the meal time is usually late, putting a strain on the digestion, which does not work at its best at night (see box, page 47). Alcohol adds to the problem, first stimulating your appetite and then adding to the calories you are taking in.

Buffet meals are a particular danger. It has been noted that, at a buffet, people put more on their plate than they should because the

WAYS IN WHICH ALCOHOL ADDS TO OUR WEIGHT

🍎 Alcoholic drinks are usually high in calories and alcohol is absorbed quickly by the body, so it spares other sugars and fats that we have eaten from being utilized as a source of energy. These are then deposited as body fat.

🍎 Wines and aperitifs increase the heart rate as they consume oxygen to get metabolized. This creates a demand for more energy and thus for food.

🍎 White wine, champagne and spirits also increase stomach acid and so stimulate appetite. Alcohol facilitates the absorption of fats (just as alcohol wipes are used to clean greasy surfaces as they absorb oils and fats very efficiently).

🍎 Liqueurs and sweet alcoholic drinks have a lot of sugar in them. Consumed at the end of a meal, these are likely to be destined to become fat deposits in the body.

🍎 A bulging 'beer belly' comes from regularly consuming excess alcohol (not just beer), which builds up fat deposits around the intestines.

variety of foods on display is an overwhelming temptation to try everything, goaded by the underlying thought that 'it may run out later'. They then eat everything on their plate, whether they actually want to or not. A vast choice and the offer to eat as much as you like for a fixed price (or, in the case of a party, for no price) is a further inducement into consuming a lot more than you need.

holidays and festivals

Holidays, whether at home or away, are typically a time for eating and drinking to excess. People in general put on weight during festive periods such as Christmas, New Year and Easter – which is ironic when Easter is supposed to be approached by a period of penance and abstinence. Supermarket shelves groan with attractive displays and manage to convey the message that it won't last long so you need to buy it now. You are therefore tempted to buy more food than you ever need, and then feel obliged to consume it rather than waste it.

Of all the types of holidays, perhaps cruises are the worst for weight gain. To have so many people trapped together in a ship is not easy. Meals are served all day long to keep passengers happy and busy, and food can easily become a main focus of the trip.

the lure of the supermarket shelves

Take-aways and supermarket ready-prepared meals – just heat and eat – tempt you to replace home-made meals: they are promoted as fast, cheap and convenient (no washing up afterwards). It's easy to go for something that cuts down the trouble of shopping, preparing, cooking and cleaning.

But there is a price to pay. Canned, preserved and precooked meals must use some form of preservative to increase shelf life. The most 'natural' of these are sugar (usually in the form of syrup) and vinegar, which of course is very acidic – most ready-to-use sauces, for instance, are either very sweet or very sharp. And so we find once again that our appetite is being manipulated by what we eat. At least you are aware of what is going into home-cooked meals and you can control the fat, sugar, salt and acid content.

Commercialism in the food industry takes no notice of people's requirements. Choice is huge, which means that competition and rivalry in the industry is high. From time to time, tailored research by food lobby-ists makes all sorts of claims that filter into the media: 'A glass of red wine a day is good for the heart'; 'Chocolate helps children's memories'; 'A glass of orange juice a day keeps cancer at bay'. They may sound like healthy advice, but the real intent is to increase sales.

What a depressing catalogue of pressures on us! Happily, however, it is quite possible to change the odds and give ourselves the upper hand in manipulating our appetite rather than allow it to manipulate us. In Chapter 10 I shall explore how we can do this.

YEASTS

Penicillin was the wonder drug of the last century. It was a fungus that killed bacteria and saved many lives. For millennia there had been an equilibrium in nature among bacteria, viruses and fungi. Within decades, penicillin and the antibiotics that followed put this peaceful co-existence to the test. Bacteria became our worst enemy and we waged a war on them with antibiotics, germ killers and antibacterial cleaning materials. Bacteria mutated and fought back, so we invented new weapons and the one-upmanship escalated. The mutant MRSA bacterium now threatens everybody who stays and works in hospitals – just the place where you hope to get better.

With bacteria being periodically battered, opportunistic fungi and viruses have multiplied and become stronger. The most common fungal infections are candida and yeast overgrowth. Until two decades ago, yeast was the natural source of vitamin B and was widely used. Today it creates a risk of thrush. Yeast and candida, a mutant form of yeast that depends on the gut wall for its nutrients, are parasites. Like worms in the intestines, they can create food cravings.

Yeast in our digestive system also ferments into alcohols, some of which are toxic. These alcohols provide the body with an easy alternative source of energy, just as an alcoholic drink would, and so more of the food we eat gets converted into fat deposits. The alcohols produced by the yeast produce a feeling of heaviness and lethargy about an hour after a meal, when alcohol concentration in the blood rises. This lethargy induces a craving for some 'instant energy' in the form of sugar, so beginning a cycle that leads to weight gain.

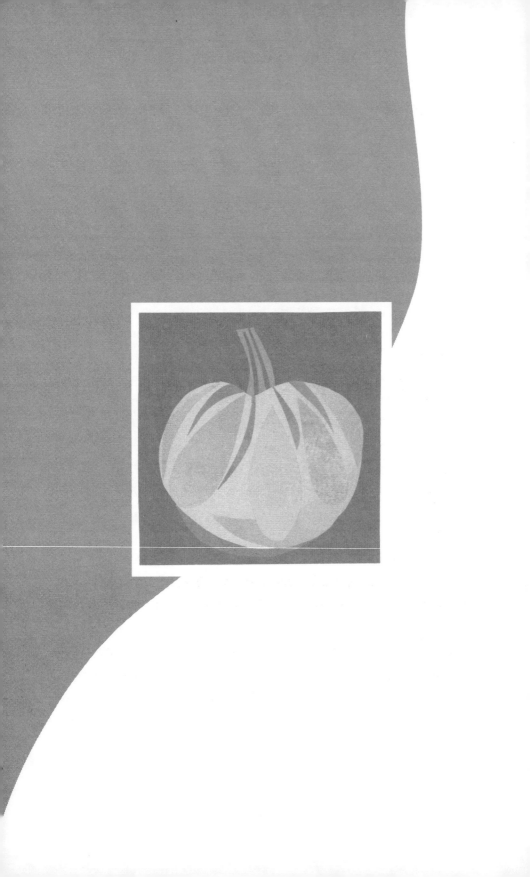

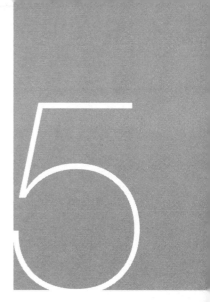

Why Does Digestion Make a Difference?

Every bit of a meal that a python swallows is digested and absorbed. Panther or tiger droppings consist of little more than their prey's hair as almost everything else is digested. Comparatively, we humans excrete far more of what we ingest. Imagine if all the food we ate, three times a day, 365 times a year, was totally absorbed. We would be enormous. Nature has protected us to some degree from this disaster by developing a digestive system that absorbs only a part of what we eat. Of the rest, some we excrete and the rest is stored as fat. If we don't use up that fat, then excess weight is the inevitable result.

If our digestion is perfectly regulated with the right quality and quantity of food, then weight gain and other health problems would be considerably reduced. All too often, though, we simply scoff down whatever we want and hope it will sort itself out. Our digestive system is vital to keeping us healthy, energetic and an appropriate weight, so it deserves our respect. Overloading the digestive system with too much or too much variety at once puts great stress on it – after the lungs of smokers, this is the most abused system in the body.

It is also useful to bear in mind that our digestive system, like the rest of our body, is much more resilient and forgiving when we are young. As we age we lose that natural robustness and so need to be much more careful. However, it is also harder to retrain and learn new habits, so it is far better to look after our digestion all along.

There are three main components to the digestive process: ingestion (eating), digestion (chemical processing as food moves from one section to the next of the digestive system) and elimination.

ingestion

As we chew our food, the saliva helps to moisten it and does some preliminary digestion of simple carbohydrates (sugars). This sugar stimulates the tastebuds to signal the brain that food is on its way.

The tastebuds also signal the brain to prepare the digestive system for what they identify: sweet, salty, bitter or sour food. Given this information, the digestive system can prepare itself and marshal the right enzymes for efficient digestion of the nutrients that will be arriving.

Eating slowly and chewing properly allows the tastebuds a chance to analyse the type and quantity of the food and helps the stomach with some preparatory work in breaking down what we have eaten. Bypassing this important analysis – by eating too fast or not chewing properly – makes the system work harder and can cause digestive problems and even difficulty in absorbing nutrients.

digestion

Everything we eat and drink is subjected to several digestive processes so that they can be absorbed and used by our bodies. Proteins are broken down into amino acids, carbohydrates into glucose, fats into lipids.

The stomach churns up what we have eaten and drunk and begins the breakdown with its powerfully acidic gastric juices. After a heavy meal, this activity draws a lot of blood to the abdominal area. This deprives the brain of blood and therefore the glucose and oxygen supply to the brain drops. This creates fatigue and a craving for sweets. That is why we so often want dessert after a meal even though the stomach is full – the appetite centre is a more powerful stimulant than receptors in the stomach.

Unlike the acid medium of the stomach, digestion in the intestines takes place in an alkaline environment. This is created by bile. The liver produces 700–1200 ml of bile a day, which should be enough to neutralize the amount of acid secreted by the stomach. But stress, eating a lot of acidic foods, eating too fast and other habits to which we are prone all increase stomach acidity (see page 35). When the stomach's contents are more acidic than they should be, digesting becomes a slow process as instead of passing quickly through to the intestines, this acidulated food has to sit in the stomach waiting for enough bile to

BAJRASANA, OR THUNDERBOLT POSE

This is a yoga posture to improve the digestive function. Kneel down and sit on your heels, with your arms folded in your lap. Keep the spine erect and close your eyes. Breathe in and out slowly and rhythmically. Maintain this position for 10 minutes.

By sitting like this after meals you reduce the blood supply to the legs and therefore make available additional blood to the digestive system when it needs it.

neutralize it. This causes acid indigestion and other discomforts. It also delays the onset of hunger because the stomach walls are stretched and the sensation of fullness continues, but that is done at a great cost.

Meats and fats take longer to digest and so suppress appetite over a longer period. Vegetables and carbohydrates are more quickly digested and if you are a strict vegetarian you may often find yourself wanting to snack on fatty or sugary foods to appease your appetite.

Keeping it simple

In my *Nutrition Bible*, I wrote about a buffet meal at which you imagine helping yourself to all the food and drinks on offer, depositing them in a bucket and stirring them up. The result is a disgusting mess of food, but that is what we expect our system to cope with.

The general rule is: the simpler the combination of foods, the better it is for the digestive system. Each food type requires different enzymes and takes a different time to digest: carbohydrates are digested the quickest, fats take longer and protein the longest time. When you load the system with all three at once, it puts the whole body under stress, especially if the quantity is large too.

If you ate a meal of lean meat, potato and three vegetables and waited an hour or so before following with some fruit, your digestive system would be delighted. Better still would be a regular regime that gave your system food to digest in combinations that it found simplest. This might be:

- porridge and toast for breakfast
- fish or chicken and salad for lunch
- pasta or rice and vegetables for dinner
- fruit eaten separately.

Your system would then have the opportunity to digest carbohydrate in the morning, protein with some fat and simple carbohydrate with roughage for lunch and carbohydrates for dinner. (If dinner is the main meal, then the day's protein with vegetables would be all right, but avoiding slow-digesting protein in the evening is preferable.)

An eating pattern like this – often called food combining – is simple for the digestive system and explains why so many people find food-combining diets beneficial to their health and weight control.

Helping the process along

Digestion also involves movement of the intestines or the bowels. Resting a while after lunch, so that there are no other major demands on your blood supply, will maximize blood flow to your abdomen and there-fore aid digestion. After dinner, walking for 5–10 minutes (even indoors if you cannot get out) will stimulate the intestines to function better as our

REST TIME

Digestion is a very strenuous and energy-consuming process. Churning food, secreting juices, moving part-digested food along the system, absorbing nutri-ents: this is all serious mechanical work from which the stomach and intestines need to rest, and night time is when most of the repair work of routine wear and tear is carried out. But involuntary muscles work automatically, so if there is food to process they must do their job, even at night. Food consumed at night is digested slowly, in phases.

You can give your digestive system a chance to rest and recuperate by:

- avoiding eating late at night
- periodic short fasts (see page 94)
- keeping food combinations simple (see opposite).

system is inclined to be sluggish in the evening. If you go to sleep immediately after eating, the food will lie there and then begin to be digested
in the early hours of the morning when the body may not need it. The
result will be more stored fat and consequently more weight gain.

elimination

Some people do not have a bowel movement for a couple of weeks
at a time, and reach the stage when even enemas do not help. This
naturally interferes with digestion and also makes the body intensify
the absorption process, leading to more fat being deposited. Chronic
constipation can result in uneliminated stools becoming hard and
adhering to the walls of the bowels. When this happens they add to
your overall weight and expand the abdomen, causing a bloated look
and discomfort.

Constipation is caused by several factors, but the main ones are
sluggish movement of the bowel muscles and a diet that doesn't
encourage regular bowel movements.

RELIEF WITH YOGA

Turtle pose – kneel and sit back on your heels. Bend forward, placing both
elbows by the sides of your knees and put your forehead on the floor. Take a deep
breath in and raise your head. Look as far up as you can while keeping your
elbows on the floor. Push your chest forwards. Hold your breath in this position
for five seconds. Slowly breathe out as you lower your head back to the floor.
Repeat five times.

Pawan mukt, or wind-relieving pose (see pages 123–4), is also very helpful in
alleviating constipation.

The following are all helpful:

- regular exercise
- yogic wind-relief poses (see box, opposite)
- plenty of water
- not rushing in the toilet
- plenty of roughage (spinach, bran flakes, figs)
- massaging the abdomen clockwise with oil each morning.

the role of the liver
in weight management

The liver is a wonderful organ. It survives a lot of beating from the rubbish we eat and drink, is bombarded with toxins, and the liver is involved one way or another in every morsel of food we eat, every drop of alcohol we drink and every pill we swallow.

Among the liver's many functions, those that have a direct relation to weight control include:

- secretion of bile. Without this most important digestive juice the pancreas could not empty its powerful and corrosive enzymes into the small intestines. Bile creates the alkaline medium in which those enzymes break down protein, carbohydrate and fat into finer particles that can easily be absorbed
- converting excess glucose into glycogen. This provides a quick-release energy reserve but any excess goes into the formation of body fat
- a healthy balance of hormones. Were the liver not to destroy excess hormones which are either secreted by the adrenal glands after they have done their jobs, or those that are taken in the form of medicine, for instance, these would accumulate and the body would become over-loaded. A poorly functioning liver is less effective at destroying excess

A SENSIBLE PRECAUTION

Precautionary notes on HRT and contraceptive pills warn against taking in cases of liver damage, but these drugs can themselves cause liver damage over a prolonged time. Give yourself periodic gaps of a month or two, to give the liver a chance to rectify the damage done to it by these medicines.

hormones and, as Chapter 3 explains, a hormonal imbalance can lead to an increase in weight that is particularly difficult to lose

 all blood passing through the intestines then passes through the liver to be detoxified before entering the main circulatory system. A liver afflicted by a disease, a tumour or cirrhosis (hardening from alcohol or infection) will block the natural flow and the result is an abdomen swollen with retained fluid.

The liver is incredibly resilient and has remarkable self-healing powers, but punishment will take its toll. Since our concern here is weight, the vital role played by the liver in weight control makes it very much in our interests to keep it healthy.

Foods to keep the liver healthy

Certain foods and herbal preparations are known to assist liver function and aid healing (in India viral jaundice is treated very effectively with herbs). Some of these include grape juice, radish, milk thistle and baby corn. The best way of keeping your liver in good shape, though, is to practise moderation in food and drink. Fasting (see Chapter 9) is a wonderful natural way of allowing it to recuperate.

the role of the kidneys in weight management

Our kidneys become involved in weight control principally in three ways:

- water retention
- protein overload
- hormonal irregularity.

Fine tubes in the kidneys filter water, waste products, excess sugar (in diabetics) and various minerals and hormones, and flush them out in the form of urine. This very necessary work can be interrupted or impaired by a number of problems, such as diabetes, kidney stones, auto-immune diseases such as lupus, urinary tract infections, congenital defects (renal cysts), drugs and alcohol abuse. Once the kidneys' filtration system suffers, fluids do not get flushed out in the normal way. A build-up of fluids results in puffiness and bloating in various parts of the body, including the legs, abdomen and face.

BE KIND TO YOUR KIDNEYS

Kidneys do not like an excess of:
- protein
- salt
- coffee
- heavy metals (found in some Chinese and Indian medicinal preparations for weight loss, sexual stimulation or energy)
- heavy-duty drugs (for cancer, auto-immune diseases)
- alcohol
- recreational drugs.

KIDNEY STONES

Help prevent kidney stones from forming by not eating an excess of red meat, shellfish, onions, tomatoes, spinach and kidney beans. (A tendency towards kidney stones can be genetic, so these precautions are especially relevant if stones are prevalent in your family).

Drinking plenty of water is the best way to flush the kidneys and help them in their work. Certain herb teas, such as nettle tea and gokhru (the dried berry from an Indian thorntree), are also effective diuretics and help with water retention.

Whereas our bodies store excess fat and carbohydrates, excess protein simply gets expelled from the system, via the kidneys. One of the complications of a high-protein diet is that the kidneys are affected by the overload (see Case Study, page 167). Sometimes kidney diseases cause protein to be lost through the urine, which can also bring on generalized water retention.

Those hormones again

Kidneys can also work against you when the wrong messages come through from the brain. The hypothalamus houses the centre that secretes a hormone called ADH (antidiuretic hormone). This hormone stops the kidneys from filtering water should the body be in danger of excessive fluid loss, for instance through acute diarrhoea or excessive heat. Sometimes this ADH centre malfunctions and the 'water retention message' doesn't switch off. The situation gets worse in very hot weather, when there may be genuine dehydration in addition to mis-interpretation and this leads to even greater fluid retention as well as great discomfort.

Aldosterone is a hormone that regulates the minerals potassium and sodium in the body, via the kidneys. In excess it causes the retention of sodium, which prevents water from being eliminated, once more causing fluid retention and adding to weight problems.

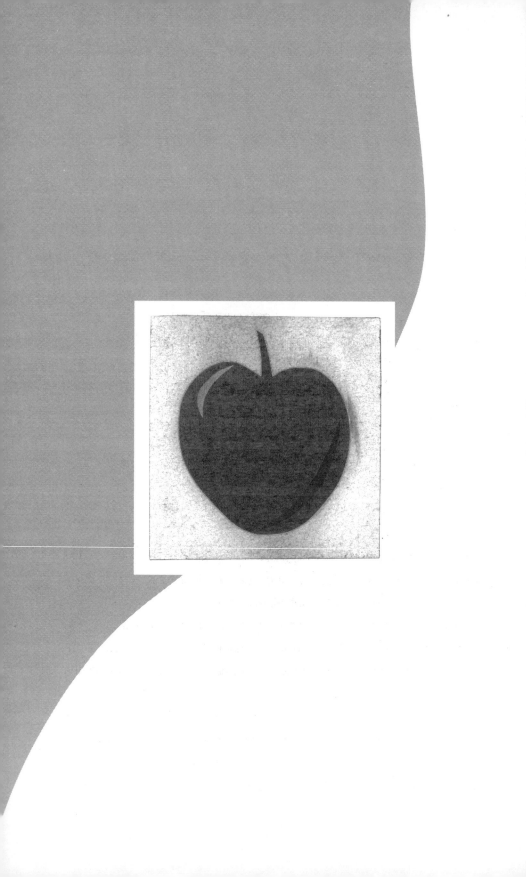

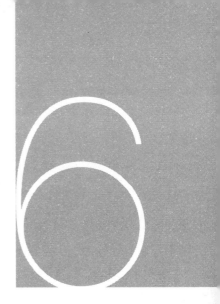

The Neck Connection

Over the past 20 or so years, I have been studying the role of a pair of arteries in the neck. These arteries originate from the major blood vessels out of the heart and pass through a bony canal formed by the cervical vertebrae and enter the skull. Tracing their pathway shows that they primarily supply blood to the subconscious part of the brain, including the pituitary and hypothalamic areas.

The subconscious part of the brain is the oldest part of the brain in terms of evolution. It deals with all the involuntary functions, such as breathing, heart rate, appetite, posture and coordination, digestion, healing, the immune system, reaction to stress, fluid retention, temperature regulation, emotions and sleep. Our conscious brain developed later and primarily deals with voluntary movements, decision-making, logic and so on. As this newer part of the brain evolved, an additional circulatory system developed, stemming from the carotid artery, which lies in the front of the neck.

THE VULNERABLE NECK

The vertebral arteries, doing their life-sustaining job of bringing nourishment (glucose and oxygen) to the subconscious part of the brain, are well protected, but the 15 cm or so of cervical spine is fragile. The vertebrae here are loosely bound and much more mobile than the rest of the spine, allowing us to move our neck and head in several different directions.

In evolutionary terms, this improved our ability to see, hear and smell, but this enhanced mobility also made our necks more susceptible to injury. Traumas at birth (including the head having to pass through a tight birth canal, forceps delivery, the umbilical cord caught around the neck and very slow or very fast 'champagne cork' births), falls, blows to the head or face, whiplash injuries and neck surgery can all cause the vertebrae in the neck to become misaligned.

The trouble does not necessarily have to begin with a sudden trauma: postural problems (particularly when sitting in front of a computer screen all day), excessive dental work, even too many pillows in bed, can also result in misalignment. Whatever the cause, when the cervical vertebrae become misaligned the vertebral canals inevitably become narrowed or twisted, and the arteries within them are bent or kinked. This reduces the blood flow to the subconscious centres of the brain.

The body can physically survive without the conscious part of the brain, as is evident with a major stroke or dementia, but a blockage of the blood supply through the vertebral arteries will reduce the ability of the basic involuntary functions that keep us alive. The more years I spend analysing the role of the subconscious brain, and the more I discover about its functions, the more I marvel at the intelligence of nature. I don't think any computer can match its perfection.

the Ali syndrome

Reduced blood flow can bring on a whole range of symptoms, from chronic fatigue, headaches and dizziness to short-term memory loss, loss of smell and taste, and reduced libido – those who have had whiplash or neck problems will identify these symptoms. From the point of view of weight control, any interference with the subconscious brain's blood flow (and therefore source of nourishment) can lead to impaired hormonal functions, fluid retention and cravings for sugary foods.

I have called the link I have established between the vertebral arteries and these symptoms the Ali Syndrome. The medical community may not accept this term as no scientific studies have been done to substantiate this hypothesis, but I have used logic and practical experience to prove retrospectively that my assumptions were correct.

For the sceptics of my hypothesis on the vertebral artery connection, I would simply point out that, when brain cells receive just marginally less blood, the brain under-functions, which results in sluggishness of

INTERESTING CONNECTIONS BETWEEN NECK INJURY AND WEIGHT GAIN

After whiplash, falls, or trauma to the head and neck, many people will put on weight.

Premenstrual tension, and particularly craving for sweets, is worse in women with a history of trauma to the neck. Before periods the blood is congested in the pelvic area, so less flows through the brain. If there is a neck connection, the depletion of blood in the brain is even greater.

Most children with traumatic birth or childhood injuries (which might be as varied as cutting the chin or falling off a swing) have symptoms of the Ali Syndrome, including food cravings and related problems such as obesity, hormonal weight gain at puberty and even bulimia.

the corresponding organs or systems in the body. When the blood supply is moderately reduced, the brain centre or cells begin to 'panic' or hyperfunction in desperation for a brief period, again altering corresponding bodily functions. When the blood supply is severely reduced, the centres collapse and can even die.

the effect on weight

The neck connection has particular importance to weight gain and loss because any reduction of blood flow can affect the functioning of the pituitary–hypothalamic area of the subconscious brain. Chapter 3 explains how the pituitary and hypothalamus regulate various hormones and the effect these have on weight.

Depriving the hypothalamus of optimum blood flow means:

🍏 the appetite centre receives less glucose, begins to panic and creates a demand for food, especially a craving for sugar

🍏 the ADH (antidiuretic hormone) centre in the hypothalamus begins to misinterpret the condition as dehydration (less blood = less fluid) and instructs the kidneys to slow down filtration, causing fluid retention.

If the blood flow to the pituitary gland is reduced, a range of hormonal weight problems can occur:

🍏 if the thyroid malfunctions there can be a massive change in weight

🍏 if the ovarian functions are affected, the body will store white fat (cellulite)

🍏 if the adrenal glands are affected and they secrete excess androgens these will be aromatized into oesterone and also result in cellulite

🍏 excess secretion of cortisol from the adrenal glands can lead to Cushing's syndrome, which manifests itself as a 'moon face' and fat redistribution together with increased appetite.

A WEALTH OF BENEFITS

Increasing the blood flow to the subconscious part of the brain via the vertebral arteries can have a positive effect on you in a number of ways.

Benefits include:

suppression of appetite and cravings: If the neck is carefully looked after and the blood flow is good, the appetite centre in the hypothalamus behaves normally. This reduces the cravings for sweets or sugar when you are tired or stressed, when you are digesting a big meal either during the afternoon or at night and before periods.

balance of hormones: Increasing the blood flow to the pituitary gland arrests the production of cellulite or white fat, although the cellulite already deposited does not shift even if the blood flow is reinstated to its full capacity. (For dealing with this, see pages 135–6.)

control of fluid retention: As the ADH centre, which controls fluid retention, receives more blood it no longer feels under threat of dehydration, and fluid retained in the body is released.

improvement in emotions and moods: The limbic system (the network of nerves in the subconscious brain) houses the centres that control emotions. Improving blood flow reduces mood swings and helps bring food cravings, comfort eating and psychological bingeing under control. I have even helped bulimics by neck manipulation and massage. (Obsessive compulsive eating, however, does not respond to the Ali technique as this is controlled by the higher centres in the conscious brain.)

a sense of well-being: As my technique helps to improve blood supply to the entire subconscious part of the brain, the whole body (and brain) feels energized as a result. Feelings of panic or depression fade, digestion and sleep improve and mood lifts. This feel-good factor makes you more aware of eating, exercising and remaining healthy, and so has an indirect but very positive effect on weight control.

It is logical that improving the blood flow to the pituitary–hypothalamic area can resolve many problems that directly or indirectly lead to weight gain. The Ali technique, which I have been using for nearly 20 years, is well known to most of my patients and readers. Conventional doctors found it absurd that by increasing the blood flow to the brain, diseases and their symptoms could be cured, but as time went by, many discovered the logical sense in it. My trainee doctors had the chance to see first-hand proof of my hypothesis and to witness the beneficial effects of the technique. Today they are successfully using the technique in their practices.

the Ali technique

The head, which is a heavy organ, is supported on the seven vertebrae of the neck and kept erect by muscles. When you fall asleep sitting up, your head drops forward as the vertebrae cannot hold the head up once the muscles relax. The muscles have to be kept toned to maintain an erect posture, but they are put under great strain by, among other things:

- insomnia
- an awkward sleeping position
- driving
- whiplash injury
- long periods in front of a computer screen

As cranial osteopaths know, the skull contracts and expands minutely about 12 times a minute in a slow, rhythmical pattern. Tight or extremely weak neck muscles will affect the circulation of cerebrospinal fluid and reduce glucose supply to the outer surface of the brain and the pituitary gland.

Massage will tone up the neck muscles, which will be sore at first, because of a build-up of lactic acid and inflammation, especially as they are put under great strain by insomnia or an awkward sleeping position, driving, whiplash injury and long periods in front of a computer screen.

In principle, the Ali technique is a massage-manipulative technique supported by therapeutic yoga. The neck is genuinely fragile, so massage should be done with care, especially when it has been operated on, or in cases of osteoporosis, severe disc prolapse and so on. Chapter 12 explains the basics of my neck massage technique and the yoga postures described in Chapter 11 also help improve blood flow in this crucial area.

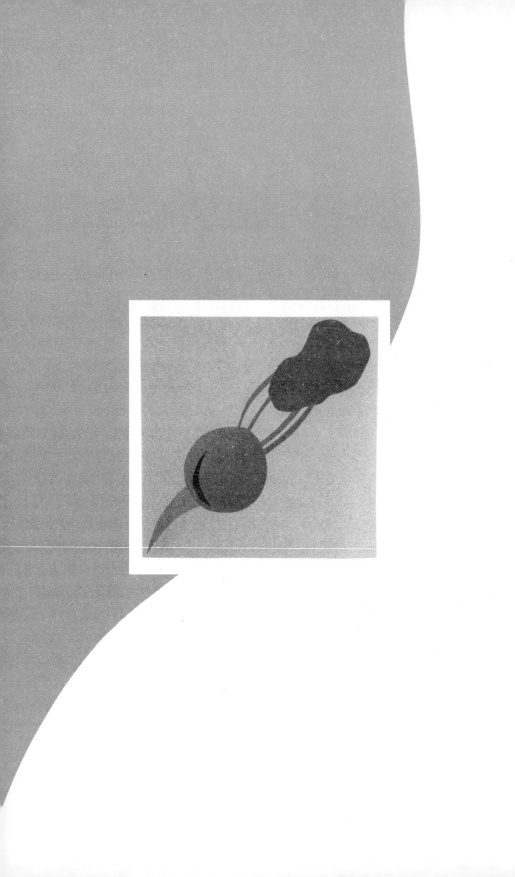

Mind Over Matter

We all recognize that alcohol, recreational drugs, even excess coffee consumption affect our behaviour, our ability to reason, our mood and inhibitions. We can also get addicted to food – chocolate, chillies, coffee and alcohol again, among others – and it is well-established that eating disorders such as bulimia, anorexia and obsessive compulsive eating have psychological components.

Even without venturing into the bounds of excess or addiction, however, some foods can have a powerful effect on the mind. Something as simple and everyday as sugar will alter our emotions and psychological behaviour. The degree of change in the mind varies from individual to individual and is affected by mentality, personality, constitution and conditions such as diabetes, liver disease or gut yeast.

The relationship between the mind and food is a close and often subtle one. Adapting the expression 'mind over matter', I say 'mind over

SUGAR POWER

Our brain cells are highly specialized but their main fuel requirements are simple: oxygen and glucose. When the level of oxygen in our blood dips, our brain feels tired and our entire body gets sluggish as if it is having a power failure. If the oxygen levels dip to an alarming level, the body goes into a panic attack in desperation – the heart beats faster and the breathing rate goes up.

When glucose levels in the blood drop our brain also feels extremely tired and craves sustenance. The appetite centre creates in us the urge to eat some sugar quickly for instant energy. A lump of sugar resolves the problem immediately. If blood sugar levels drop drastically the body reacts alarmingly, as diabetics know when they suffer from hypoglycaemia: a sinking feeling, cold sweats, extreme fatigue, nausea and faintness.

With excess consumption of sugar, the opposite occurs and our brain becomes overactive. With it comes irritability and agitation. We all know that children who eat a lot of sweets are inclined to be hyperactive, sometimes to the extent of losing all control. If you eat a very sweet dessert at night you may find your mind becomes active and it is difficult to get to sleep.

To complicate matters further, if you suffer from candida, a gut yeast problem (see page 41), the sugar you ingest is turned into a form of alcohol in your system, which makes you very heady and often very lethargic.

matter is matter undermined': by recognizing and capitalizing on this relationship we can use it to our own benefit.

appreciating food

Traditionally, in regions of the world from China and India to the Middle East and Europe, a meal time was a regular opportunity for the family to gather together, discussing the food and enjoying it. Prayers beforehand underlined a sense of appreciation and thankfulness. It was a special occasion.

Today, it is much rarer for the immediate family, let alone extended families, to sit down frequently to eat together in this way. More often than not, everyday eating is something squeezed between other activities, and the mind is not focused on food. Then, at social gatherings too much food is eaten, and alcohol removes the inhibition to overeat, so it is only when stomach walls are fully stretched and feeling uncomfortable that we realize we have eaten too much. And even then, we may not be able to say what exactly it is we have swallowed and what it tasted like.

You will read more than once in this book: eat slowly – and I make no apologies for repeating it again here. If you eat quickly, without paying any attention, you are disengaging your mind from the food. Bring your brain back into the equation and it will stop you overeating and improve your digestion. As explained in Chapter 4, let your taste-buds appreciate what you are eating, and the messages they send, via your brain, will enable the appetite centre to send 'full' signals in plenty of time. My grandfather, who was a doctor–homeopath, used to say: 'Stop eating when you think another mouthful will make you full.' In other words, listen to the tell-tale signs of the body to restrict the volume of food you consume. Eating slowly is a habit – and forming the right eating habits is essential for weight control.

I also recommend approaching meals in the right frame of mind. Prayers are said before eating in many religions. In traditional Indian families, the standard ritual was to sprinkle some water with your hands and say a prayer before eating. It concentrated your mind on the meal to come and made you mindful of both waste and gluttony. The Christian 'Lord's Prayer' includes the very appropriate words: 'Give us this day our daily bread ...'; '... and lead us not into temptation ...'. What a wonderful reminder that a regular supply of food is something to be grateful for, and should not be abused. Meals need not be prefaced by a formal prayer, but it is very helpful to set aside a moment to reflect on the gift of food, on the world's starving millions and to give thanks – even a minute or two of contemplation makes overeating harder.

the senses

Never underestimate the part all our senses play in our relationship with food. Apart from taste, the smell of food has an obvious impact on appetite, and the two senses work closely together. Those who lose their sense of smell or suffer from burning mouth syndrome find their sense of taste is also impaired.

🍎 ***The eyes*** also play an important role. Our salivary glands, even our stomach, can react to the sight of a rich creamy cake or a half-rotten lettuce even before the other senses have had a chance to collect any information. We have learnt to have certain expectations of what food should look like, and would probably shy away from a blue apple even if it was harmlessly coloured and tasted no different to a green one. A recent survey by Indian restaurants found that customers were not ordering tandoori chicken or tikka masala unless artificial red colouring was added, because that was what they had come to expect. Accomplished cooks, whether professional or not, know that food that looks appetizing on the plate is going to be more highly appreciated than an amorphous, mono-coloured serving. 'Eating with our eyes' can play havoc with our stomachs.

🍎 ***Touch*** is perhaps a more surprising contributor to our perception of food, but the fingers are amazing sensory organs. Traditionally, in India, Africa and the Middle East, people use their hands to eat. It certainly gives more satisfaction than eating with utensils. While mixing food on the plate, some signals are perhaps sent to the brain that add to the tastebuds' signals from the tongue, and so with spoons, forks or

A few years aso, I took a group of doctors to Oman to give an introductory course in homeopathy, acupuncture, yoga and ayurveda to medical students. We were invited to a friend's house to meet a group of blind youths who had been trained in Indonesia to 'see' and 'taste' with their hands. Besides riding a bicycle, they could 'read' colours and could differentiate pulverised sugar from salt, both of which feel and look the same to a sighted person. Fingers have extraordinary powers of perception.

chopsticks one runs a greater risk of eating more. Grinding or feeling the smoothness of food adds value to the taste and satisfaction derived from food, and people with dentures or implants often find they cannot taste their food as well as they did with natural teeth. As a result they have a tendency to eat more in the search to feel full or satisfied.

the conditioned reflex

The conditioned reflex identified by the Nobel prize-winning physiologist Ivan Pavlov is well known. Before he fed the dogs in his laboratory, he would ring bells and flash lights, and the dogs soon learnt that these signals preceded a meal. Then, the same dogs received the signals but no food. Their excitement, salivation and gastric juice secretion were identical. These animals had been conditioned to associate certain signals with food, and their brains sent out the same anticipatory reflexes whether or not food actually appeared.

We may think that, being capable of rather greater reasoning than dogs, our bodies do not react to basic stimuli like this. But they do. Just before lunchtime, most people get a sense of being hungry, their stomach acid secretion increases and they get slightly irritated. We are conditioned to mealtimes. And we should not ignore these reflexes because they gear up the body to receive and digest food and we should take advantage of this. Sticking to fixed times for meals is excellent for the digestion – if you skip a meal you will probably be very hungry by the next one, so you will eat quickly and eat more. Or you will snack in between meals but still feel you 'should' eat at the next meal, because you are conditioned to do so. This conditioning is one of the things that makes jet lag so tiresome until your body has adjusted to the new time zone.

Having said that, you should eat when you are hungry, but don't make yourself eat if you are not, just to keep to a timetable. If, after a heavy dinner, you feel you cannot eat breakfast in the morning, so be it. Forcing yourself to eat breakfast then would be an error as that food may be more than your body needs and will get deposited as fat.

think before you eat

In short, you have to apply your mind when you eat. This is something that you need to develop, and for some, bad habits may be deeply ingrained and need a lot of concentration to overcome. It's not easy. Since we no longer have to hunt for our food, and there is so much, so readily available, we are in danger of taking it for granted – it is possible even to forget that someone somewhere must have participated in its making. Regaining respect for food, understanding its effects, learning to appreciate it with all your senses and engaging your brain in the eating process leads to a much healthier approach to food and is of enormous assistance in long-term weight loss. Here are some tips:

 fasting from time to time makes you much more highly aware of the effect food has on you mentally as well as physically

 refrain from certain specific foodstuffs for a period and gauge how you feel. Try a month without one or more of the following: yeast, coffee, alcohol. To test yourself, see how differently you feel after a cup of coffee or a couple of sandwiches after your period of abstinence. You may feel quite unwell – think about what your body might be telling you. You can get used to that specific food again, but practise moderation

🍎 a minute of silence, either in prayer or contemplation, before a meal helps you to apply your mind to what you are eating and how much you eat

🍎 eat slowly to help your body make its own judgements about what and how much you eat

🍎 teach your children good food habits when they are young. Making changes may be hard for you, but you can make the future easier for them

🍎 yoga, exercise and meditation all help give you new respect for your body and your mind as well as improving your well-being.

THE POWER OF POSITIVE THINKING

Before you go on a dietary plan to lose weight you must motivate yourself:

'I want to be healthy; this excess weight can affect my health and I must get rid of it. The new regime of diet and exercise is good for me. I must follow the plan. I want to fit into my clothes again. By looking good, I want to feel good.'

Repeat this thought several times a day, particularly when you get ready to eat or exercise.

Part Two

The Weight Loss Plans

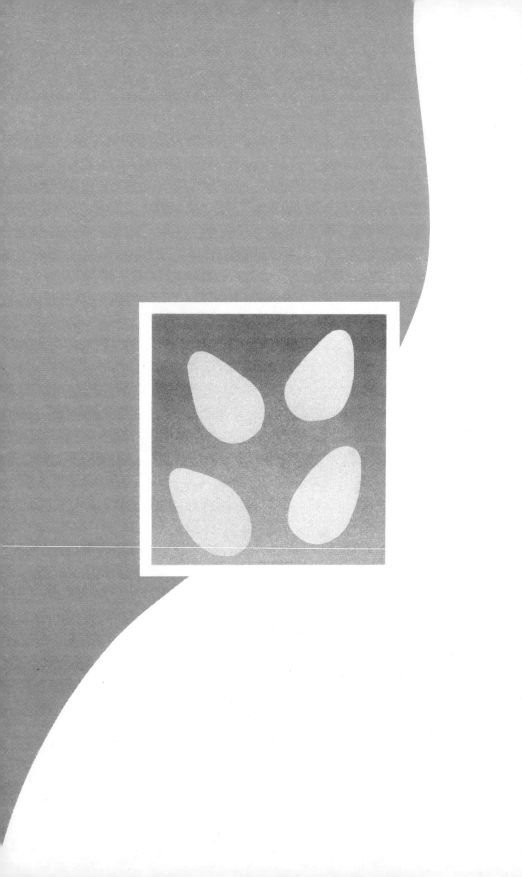

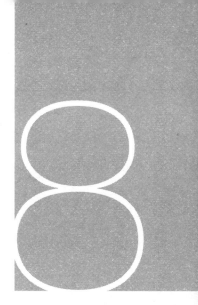

Self-
assessment

You will have realized by now that being overweight can stem from a number of different causes, and that how you set about losing weight will depend on the cause – what is right for one person is not necessarily right for another.

You may already have a shrewd idea of the reason for your excess weight, but working through the questions on the following pages and giving them honest consideration will help you to decide on your personal best route to a healthy weight. How you answer them will help you to determine the principal cause of your being overweight. This is not a competitive text – so there is no point in fudging or guessing your answers – but a way of highlighting points for you to consider, and perhaps to throw new light on the way your body is working, or not working, for you.

Questions to ask yourself 1

Do you find that you lose weight if:

🍎 you go on a simple diet, such as food combining, cabbage soup diet for a week, low-fat diet, vegetarian diet, etc?

🍎 you restrict yourself to a fruit-only breakfast and light lunches and dinners of salads and soups (for example in hot weather)?

🍎 you give up specific high-calorie items such as alcohol, bread, butter or cream?

🍎 you go on a walking or activity holiday?

🍎 you take up a regular exercise regime, such as swimming, jogging, tennis or an aerobic exercise class?

🍎 you undertake a two- or three-day fast or a period of semi-fasting (such as during Lent or Ramadan)?

🍎 you lose your appetite for a period (perhaps from a minor ailment not related to food, or during a time of bereavement)?

Do you find that as soon as you stop any of the above, you put the weight back on again?

If you answer Yes to at least some of these questions, you are typical of most people. The problem is getting the right balance between energy intake and energy expenditure – i.e. you put on weight when you eat more than you burn off, and you lose weight when you use up more than you eat.

Chapter 13 describes the appropriate weight loss plan for you, and Chapters 9 (Fasting), 10 (Regulating What You Eat) and 11 (Therapeutic Yoga and Exercise) will also prove very helpful.

If you could not answer Yes to any of the above, continue with the next set of questions.

Questions to ask yourself 2

🍎 If you follow a strict diet regime, do you find the results are neglible?

🍎 Do you eat very sensibly and still continue to gain weight?

🍎 Does your excess fat particularly accumulate on the sides of the thighs, below the tummy button, around the breast area, on the upper arms and on the buttocks/hips?

🍎 Do you have stretch marks over your fattest parts?

🍎 Was there anything at your birth that might have caused an injury to the skull or neck (a forceps/ventouse delivery, ultra-rapid birth, delayed birth of over 24 hours)?

🍎 Did you have any injuries in childhood that cut your head, broke your nose or a fall that knocked you unconscious?

🍎 Have you put on weight after taking steroids for over three months?

🍎 Do you take thyroxine because of a low thyroid function?

🍎 Did you start putting on weight at puberty?

Questions for women

🍎 Have your periods ever stopped or become irregular or scant (apart from at the menopause)?

🍎 Have you taken or did you take the contraceptive pill or HRT for more than two years?

🍎 Do you suffer from endometriosis?

🍎 Do you have polycystic ovaries or small ovaries (which you would probably only learn about after medical investigation)?

🍎 Have you put on weight after a hysterectomy?

🍎 Do you have evidence of male-pattern hair growth?

🍎 Have you had a prolonged period of stress? (Such stress can sometimes affect hormone levels.)

Questions for men

(You may find that some of these questions are sensitive and perhaps embarrassing, but you should be honest.)

🍎 Have you developed breasts or do you have excess fat deposits in the breast area, or do you have a family history of gynaecomastia (see pages 27 and 77)?

🍎 Did your testicles not descend into the scrotum in childhood?

🍎 Have you had any infection or inflammation in the testicles?

🍎 Have you had any surgery on the testicles?

🍎 Have you suffered from an enlarged scrotum, filled with fluid (hydrocele)?

🍎 Have you had any injury to the scrotum or testicles?

If you answer Yes to any of the gender-specific questions or more than half the general questions, then your excess weight is likely to be attributable to hormones.

Contrary to what many people think, hormonal weight gain is the effect of a condition that has very little to do with diet and exercise. The weight just creeps up due to hormonal imbalances and is a defensive mechanism that is intended to help the body in a crisis situation (see Chapter 3). But this side effect has heavy cosmetic and social implications. Parents often criticize their teenage children for being fat and it can cause huge loss of self-confidence and great marital discord. You might expect a hormone problem to show up in blood tests. However, thyroid tests or oestrogen level tests do not always measure any abnormality. This is because hormones keep fluctuating as the body's requirements vary, and a borderline situation may be difficult to catch. Also, low thyroid hormones cause only a percentage of weight gain; excess weight is also due to the conversion of androgens into oesterone in white cellulite fat, and their levels may not be recorded as raised.

MEN CAN HAVE PROBLEMS TOO

It is generally women who suffer from hormone-related weight gain but, as you will have seen from the questions above, many men are affected too. If you have had any problems with the testicles or scrotum, including hernia into the scrotum, the chances are that there would be some complications with testicular functions. A less usual situation is that, if it had not been detected early on that your testicles had not descended properly, or no action was taken, this would lead to feminization of the body. This can result in breast development, cellulite deposits, etc., and often infertility. Such a hormonal imbalance can affect your weight and fat distribution.

A simple diagnosis is to stand naked before a mirror and see where the specific areas of fat deposits are. If they are noticeably around the buttocks, thighs and belly, giving you a pear shape, rather than the more common round 'apple' shape that overweight men develop, and if you have the appearance of breasts, then you know that hormones are at the base of your problem.

Gynaecomastia, the development of glandular breast tissue (see page 27), is not a result of being overweight but has a bearing on your weight and effective control of it. Because it is hormonal in origin and indicates an upset in the hormonal balance, it is a condition that can also be accompanied by a tendency to deposits of white fat. This swelling of male breasts can also be a hereditary trait (it often happens around puberty and does not always persist), and you may find fathers, uncles or grandfathers also had it, even if it was not admitted or talked about. As well as hormonal and genetic factors, the condition also has a psychological aspect, as distress and embarrassment over your body image can lead to an altered relationship with food.

If after reading this section you find that your weight problem is hormonal in nature, Chapter 14 describes the recommended weight loss plan for you, and you should also read Chapter 3 (All About Hormones) and Chapter 6 (The Neck Connection).

genetic and familial influences

 Were your grandparents and parents obese? (At least one from each generation should have been overweight for a Yes answer to this.)

 Have you had a weight problem since childhood? (Family photos may be a help here.)

 Did you start gaining weight at puberty?

 Are your children overweight too?

It has long been recognized that fat runs in families. But is this an inescapable fact of life, like red hair or blue eyes, or is it the effect of bad eating or overeating down the generations? Are you fat because your mother was fat and her mother before her, or because you were fed too much of the wrong sorts of foods as a child and your family was not 'into' sport or exercise?

Our genetic make-up can certainly affect our weight and our efficiency to use up energy (see Chapter 1), but when excess weight runs in the family, it is probably from a mixture of causes that may be hormonal, psychological and diet-related as well as genetic in origin.

If 50 per cent or more of your family are overweight, at least part of your weight problem probably lies with family traits, whether genetic or habitual. From your answers to the questions in the earlier sections you will have determined whether your weight is basically hormonal or diet/exercise-related, but Chapter 15 will give you additional advice on overcoming the 'family link'.

psychological factors

 Do you tend to eat more when you are unhappy?

 Do you turn to food as a comfort in times of stress or from boredom?

 Do you find you cannot say No to cravings for a particular food, such as chocolate or alcohol?

🍎 Have you been diagnosed with an eating disorder such as bulimia or obsessive compulsive eating?

Of course, these are not at all of the same degree or magnitude, but an inclination to turn to food in times of stress is, in a mild form, a manifestation of a problematic relationship with food. Recognizing the cause of your cravings, whether they are regular or occasional, will help you take avoiding action.

As pages 67–8 explains, we are creatures of habit and respond to conditioned reflexes. You may find that one of the difficulties with losing weight stems from something you are doing without even thinking about it. Analysing your eating patterns more closely could identify habits that may be contributing to your weight problem.

🍎 Do you always finish everything on your plate? Is this from hunger, or from habit, or because you were taught it was polite?

🍎 Have you got in the routine of finishing up the children's leftovers?

🍎 Do you always have some cake or biscuits with coffee or tea, just out of habit rather than asking yourself whether you are hungry?

🍎 Is your evening meal the main meal of the day? Does it have to be?

🍎 Do you eat late in the evening because that is the only opportunity, or could the routine be altered?

Chapter 16 deals mainly with strategies to help cope with deep psychological difficulties such as uncontrolled eating, but also has advice on how to make more minor adjustments. Chapter 7 (Mind Over Matter) explains how what we eat influences our mind as well as our body, in ways that can be both good and bad.

some further considerations

If you have quit smoking ... Most smokers find that they put on weight as soon as they give up, which is very dispiriting. Begin on the weight loss plan outlined in Chapter 13 as soon as you give up, and include the yoga breathing exercises in Chapter 11 to improve the health of your lungs.

If you are worried about puppy fat ... Weight gain around puberty is very common and usually hormone-related. There may also be familial and psychological factors to consider. See Chapter 15 for advice on overweight teenagers.

A weight problem that has arisen in old age or around retirement? Some women put on weight after taking HRT for many years, but for most people who face an increase in weight around this time the problem is one of maintaining eating habits and amounts that are no longer appropriate. Are you over 60 but eating the same as you did at 30? Are you as active? Is your digestion as robust? As we age we need to adjust our diet to the requirements of our body. Chapter 15 includes information on eating requirements for different members of the family.

MIXED MESSAGES

Having read through this section, you may feel that your weight stems from a little bit of all these causes! It is entirely possible that you could be overweight because hormonal problems have made you reluctant to exercise and have encouraged you to turn to food for comfort. Or that the extra fat that you always assumed was an inherited feature could also be fuelled by hormones. In this case it is best to follow the plan for hormone-related overweight (Chapter 14), but take into account any relevant advice in Chapters 15 and 16 too.

body types

All the assessment so far in this section has been concerned with how your body processes what you eat and your mental relationship with food. Another aspect of self-assessment, however, is your body type. Determining this will provide further clues to your body's strengths and weaknesses and highlight where your particular difficulties may lie. And most importantly, once you have succeeded in losing weight, it can be your guide in maintaining your new self.

The fact that we are not all the same was known to humankind for thousands of years. Why modern medicine has completely ignored this is a wonder. Science has broken everything into parts and studied them individually but never all together as a whole. This has been the greatest blunder that medicine has made.

Some people can eat as much as they like and not put on any weight at all while others complain that they continue to gain weight, however little they consume. This is all part of our genetic make-up and can be classified in a number of ways. For centuries, physicians, morphologists, philosophers and others have attempted to categorize people into groups.

The Greek physician-surgeon Galen (AD 131–200) was the first recorded person to categorize people into types according to the dominance of different fluids of 'humours': sanguine (blood), choleric (yellow bile), phlegmatic (phlegm) and melancholic (black bile). He was a genius who studied the body, its functions, its diseases and its nature very deeply. He gave many organs and their diseases the names we still use – appendicitis, tonsillitis, gastritis, etc., and he described the chambers of the eye, noticing the phenomenon of inverted vision. His Caesarean sections saved many imperial children.

About 700 years later Avicenna, a remarkable Persian–Arab physician, enlarged upon Galen's basic concept of four humours (see table on page 82). Several qualities of a physical and psychological nature

ASTHEMIC OR APOPLECTIC?

For over 2,000 years ayurvedic masters have grouped people as either vata, pitta or kapha, and Hippocrates referred to apoplectic, phlegmatic and phthisical types. Pavlov labelled different people he observed as lively, impetuous, calm or weak, and in the mid-twentieth century popular groupings included mesomorph, ectomorph and endomorph or athletic, cerebral, phlegmatic and asthemic. Blood groups, rib cage shape and psychological outlook as well as physical shape have all been used for classification.

were perceived as characteristic of each type, but it is important to differentiate here between constitution and temperament.

The constitution can be defined briefly as the physical characteristics of a person. It is something that does not change much as it is genetically determined. It is the matrix of the body. Temperament is the dynamic part of a personality, taking into account the characteristics that may change as the body matures and adapts to new environments.

A physician trained in using these types as a diagnostic aid will examine a patient using all five senses and take note of general physique, pulse, feel of the skin, type of hair, sleep and work patterns, emotional characteristics, colour of stools and urine and several other characteristics. However, the following notes and table may help you to identify your underlying type.

Sanguine: Typically, sanguine people eat and digest well, can burn fat easily and have a personality that leaves no room for bingeing or other psychological conditions that may lead to weight gain. However, they can encounter weight problems. When these occur, they are likely to be through outside influences such as a working or social life that involves a great deal of eating, or an upbringing that has encouraged overeating or laziness.

Choleric: A choleric person often has digestive problems such as acid indigestion, bloating, periodic diarrhoea alternating with constipation and general abdominal discomfort. They are inclined to eat carefully but there is always the desire to try out new things. They may take antacids, herbal remedies and see many doctors, but digestion will always be a weakness. Choleric people do not easily put on weight, perhaps because digestive problems cause malabsorption of nutrients.

Phlegmatic: Phlegmatics are typically the FFF (fat, fair and flabby) type, for whom weight is always a problem. They may worry about this and try different diets, but often without much success. This is partly because much of the problem may be hormonal and partly because they have a tendency to secret bingeing or snacking that they may deny. Phlegmatics have strong likes and dislikes but, faced with their favourite foods, find it hard to control themselves. This inability to resist temptation means that they will quickly polish off any food lying around in the fridge. They often derive great enjoyment from cooking for friends and family, and when out shopping always end up buying more food than they need. Phlegmatics come across as happy-go-lucky types and great company, but deep within them are insecurities that can lead to comfort eating. If your disposition is phlegmatic, follow the dietary plan recommended in Chapter 14, but take particular note of the advice in Chapters 15 and 16.

Melancholic: Melancholics are often poor eaters and constitutionally do not tend to put on any weight. However, as they are inclined to pessimism, they are always worried about their health. They often become hypochondriacs, reading up on the illnesses they worry about. This may lead them to follow a variety of dietary programmes or they might become vegans or strict vegetarians. Since weight gain is not a common problem, melancholics should make sure that they eat enough and receive sufficient nourishment, or other health problems will ensue.

	Sanguine hot and wet (as if blood dominates)	Choleric hot and dry (as if bile dominates)
Skin feels	warm and moist	warm and dry
Fat and flesh beneath the skin feels	firm – more flesh than fat	medium – equal flesh and fat
Hair	thick and straight	thick/excessive, curly, grows quickly
Skin tone*	ruddy or rosy	sallow
Body build	muscular	medium
Reaction to climatic temperature	becomes restless in heat, sweats a lot	overheats in hot, dry (desert-type) weather
Metabolism	good pulse rate (70–80); energetic. Good appetite and digestion with regular bowel movements	good pulse rate (70–80). Good appetite and bowel movements; high stomach acid, giving indigestion/gas
Excretion	strong-smelling urine and stools	dark stools; straw-coloured urine
Sleep and wakefulness	sound sleeper (asleep as soon as head hits pillow). Wakes early, refreshed. Energy to work non-stop all day	often disturbed nights, but can go long time without sleep. Less tired at night, when mind very alert
Activity	talks fast, blinks frequently; can be hyperactive or fidgety	moves and talks quickly; tires quite easily
Moods and reactions	volatile: quick to anger but quick to cool down, without ill-feelings. Eats fast. Passionate, laughs 'from the bottom of the heart'. Makes friends easily and always cheerful. Has leadership qualities and is centre-stage in a group. Very caring. Speaks loudly. Typically optimistic.	reacts fast to emotions but cannot unwind or forget things easily. Listens rather than talks, but speaks thoughtfully and thinks deeply. Always calculating the next move. Often selfish and demanding

*Avicenna noticed that colour of skin due to geographical location or race may camouflage the true temperament.

Phlegmatic cold and wet (as if phlegm dominates)	Melancholic cold and dry (as if black bile dominates)
cold and moist	cold and dry
soft (in shorthand, FFF – fat, fair and flabby)	medium – equal flesh and fat
scanty, thin	thin, slow-growing
fair, wheatish	pale
inclined to fat	slim or thin
feels unwell in cold, wet weather, finds it hard to keep warm	worst in clear, cold weather; cold hands and feet and feels miserable
slow pulse rate (60–70); inclined to tiredness and low blood pressure. Good appetite but sluggish digestion and poor bowel movements	sluggish pulse (50–60); low blood pressure and often tired. Poor appetite, sluggish bowels, poor digestion
light-coloured urine and stools	small amounts of stools and urine
likes afternoon siesta as well as a lot of sleep at night; angered if sleep is disturbed	sleeps badly (can lay awake at night worrying); feels tired during day and will catnap on journeys or in front of TV
seemingly active but takes time to do things	speech slow and weak; does everything sluggishly
very emotional, shy, has many fears. Hesitant to speak own mind. Difficulty in expressing deeper feelings (hides grief). Spiritually inclined. Great believer in destiny and luck	Pessimistic; always afraid of mishaps or disasters; smiles with great difficulty. Broods over things; yawns a lot. Inclined to dwell in the past or the future rather than live for the present. Likely to blame himself or herself for everything

a target to aim at

It is much better to set yourself a specific target, rather than just a vague thought such as 'I want to be slimmer' or 'I want to look like Elle McPherson/Brad Pitt'. Check your Body Mass Index (see below) and work out how much you need to lose to reach an appropriate weight for your height.

Remember that actual weight can sometimes be deceptive, since muscle development and weight distribution play a part, so measure yourself too. Then, when you reach a plateau in your weight loss, you can see that your waist or thighs are still shrinking even if the scales are not showing any further reduction.

YOUR BMI

The most widely used formula for relating height and body weight is the Body Mass Index (BMI) which is:

weight in kg divided by height in metres squared

Weight should be without clothes, and height without shoes.

Here are a couple of examples of the calculation:

57 kg $\div$ 1.6 m^2 = 57 $\div$ 2.56 = 22.2
100 kg $\div$ 1.85 m^2 = 100 $\div$ 3.42 = 29.2

A BMI between 20 and 25 is considered normal for most individuals. Overweight is defined as between 25 and 27, and obesity is over 27.

The chart opposite, known as a nomogram, is a simple way of ascertaining your BMI. Read off your BMI where the ruler crosses the central scale.

NOMOGRAM

Place a ruler or other straight edge between your body weight in kilograms or pounds on the left and your height in centimeters or in inches on the right.

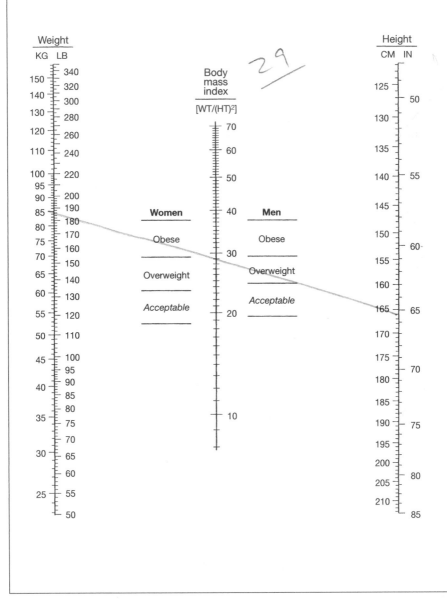

Weight

KG LB

Body
mass
index

$[WT/(HT)^2]$

Height

CM IN

Women

Obese

Overweight

Acceptable

Men

Obese

Overweight

Acceptable

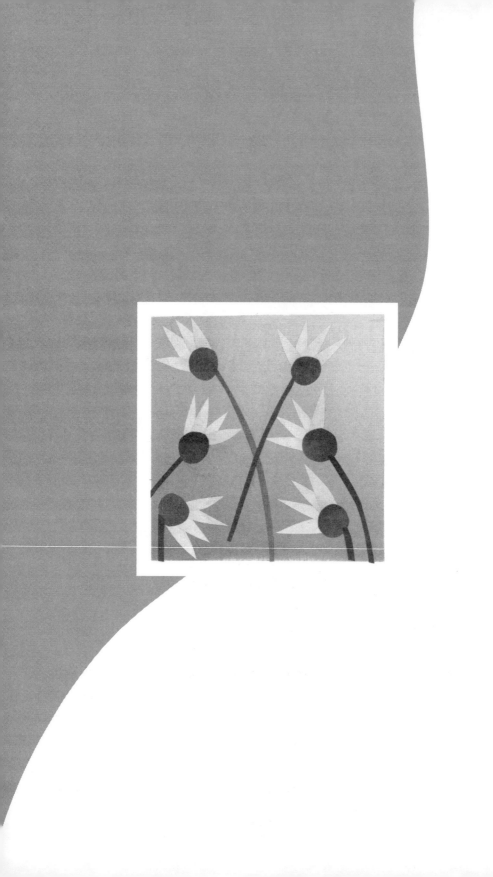

Fasting

It is obvious that if we ate three sensible meals a day, every day of our life, our body would adapt to the regime and do its best to keep us healthy. Unfortunately, we put our systems under strain by eating too much, eating at the wrong times and eating too many different foods at once. It is rare now to meet someone who eats a perfect diet. It has become essential, therefore, to look to abstinence and fasting as methods of giving our system a rest, particularly when there is a health issue such as excess weight adding to the stress put on the body.

We are conditioned to our mealtimes. As a mealtime approaches, acid secretion increases and our appetite builds up. If no food is supplied, we are likely to get angry and irritable more easily. Skipping a meal or two can cause great tension, headaches, weakness and even a sinking feeling. Probably everyone at some stage or another has experienced this. It is this fear of starving or collapsing from hunger that scares people off fasting. Yet we also know, from news stories of people surviving days under rubble after an earthquake or other disaster, that we can survive without food for quite a long time. I was in a Buddhist monastery in the Nubhra Valley, high in the Himalayas, where a monk had lived in a closed room, meditating and eating one simple meal a day, for 12 years. I also met a Jain *muni* (priest) who fasted for 60 days on nothing but water.

the fasting tradition

Most traditional religions, including Islam, Hinduism, Jainism, Buddhism, Judaism and Christianity, advocate fasting at various times. Fasting is viewed not only as a method of observing sacrifice or penance but also as a means of purification of the body and soul, and it is recognized that fasting is important for improving the healing power within the body. Hinduism and Islam have looked at the matter of fasting very deeply and have made it compulsory to observe the rituals associated with it.

Two important Hindu fasts are the seasonal Navratri fasts, one in the springtime and the other in autumn. These are times of the year when people generally tend to get ill and perhaps these fasts awaken their bodies and help them adjust to the new season. These are times for prayers and chanting, and people eat just one meal a day, at sunset, consisting of fruit, grains and some vegetables, cooked simply. There

THE RUSSIAN EXPERIENCE

My knowledge of fasting therapy began with Professor Yuri Sergeivitch Nikolaev, the great Soviet expert in this area. He treated various problems with fasting, of which the most common was obesity. In 1981 there was at least a six-month wait for admission on to the 60-bed ward that he ran. People saw the results and wanted to try it.

When I worked with Professor Nikolaev, the patients on the ward routinely fasted for two to three weeks. The psychological build-up is extremely important.

Every patient had a detailed consultation, was explained the process and benefits and was advised to go on a trial run for a couple of days with water and honey only, before they were admitted.

In most naturopathic centres fasting is done with slightly sweetened water with a few drops of lime or lemon juice in it drunk throughout the day. Professor Nikolaev recommended weak dried blackcurrant tea (4 tbsp of dried blackcurrants infused in 2 litres of boiling water for an hour). He said the blackcurrants released fructose as well as vitamin C, which is essential.

Several of Professor Nikolaev's students undertook PhD theses looking at the biochemical, physiological, psychological and social aspects of fasting. I have seen the pictures of the stomach lining in different stages taken by endoscopic cameras. The gut lining produces a thick greyish mucus in the period up to the end of the healing crisis around the ninth day (see page 99), when the discharge increases. After that, the mucus becomes clear and the lining is pink and jelly-like, comparable to the gut of a newborn baby. Professor Nikolaev explained that the mucus from the lining of the gut carried toxins and was reabsorbed, minus the toxins. In other words, in times of nutritional deprivation even the mucus discharge is reabsorbed with the help of digestive juices.

Professor Romashoff, the dean of the medical faculty where I studied in Moscow, was a student of Professor Nikolaev. He was an eminent heart surgeon but his passion lay in traditional medicine, including iridology, tongue diagnosis, yoga and fasting. Parallel to the surgical ward was a small ward where he treated thrombophlebitis, inflammation of the veins due to a blood clot, and deep vein thrombosis (such as has become familiar from stories about the dangers of not moving around during long-haul flights). In his treatment of heart disease he used fasting to remove plaque in the arteries of the heart. He proved that, during fasting, the same enzymes that reduce fat in the body dissolve these clots and restore full circulation. The clots dissolved like limescale in pipes and there was no risk of them travelling up the bloodstream to the lungs or elsewhere.

are also weekly one-day fasts dedicated to various gods, to thank them and to improve the quality of life.

Although these fasts are observed strictly for religious reasons, they have an effect on health too – this weekly pause helps keep weight in check and gives the system a chance to rectify any damage caused directly by diet. Of course, everything should be done in moderation, and unfortunately there are some zealous people, women in particular, who overdo the fasting, often when they are unhappy or there is a problem in the family. They follow every fast there is and consequently suffer from poor nutrition. One has to be cautious of such fasts, as anything in excess is bad.

Jains go further still. Because they believe in not harming any living creature, they follow a strictly vegan diet and during the monsoon season, when a lot of insects are found in fruit and vegetables, they eat nothing fresh at all, and survive on grains, lentils and dried beans. Jain priests are known to fast for a month or so at a stretch, taking in nothing more than water. To suppress their appetite and control hunger pangs they suck cloves, as clove oil numbs the nerve endings.

Sometimes, fasting becomes a practice followed to the letter but not in spirit. The Islamic fasting month of Ramadan, when nothing is eaten or drunk between sunrise and sunset, was formulated to give the body a total rest, the day's fast prepared for by a breakfast of dates and other fruit and broken by a light evening meal. Unfortunately, for some, it has become a time to sleep all day, and eat and party all night. Thus this admirable month-long fast is becoming increasingly unhealthy. And then, soon after Ramadan, comes a festive season, when all the goodness achieved during fasting is ruined.

before you fast

Before I explain the process of fasting, I must stress that longer fasts – for a period that exceeds seven days – should only be done under supervision in a medical institution. At home, you can safely go on a seven-day fast provided you are mentally prepared and have had an initial consultation with a naturopath or doctor who can guide you properly.

NATURE'S WAY

Naturopathy, nature's cure, is a practice that relies on fasting, massage, juices, saunas, hydrotherapy and other non-invasive and natural treatments – it adheres to the concept of following the rules of nature. We can see this principle at work in the wild – when animals are ill, they do not eat but you can see them drink water and eat herbs that they intuitively feel would help them. Nearer to our own experience, you may have noticed that a sick baby loses its appetite and refuses to eat other than to drink fluids.

You should not allow children to fast. Do not fast if you are pregnant or suffer from any of the following:

- diabetes
- heart disease
- epilepsy
- anaemia
- very low blood pressure (below 50 diastolic)
- kidney failure
- osteoporosis
- gout (the pain increases with fasting)
- stomach ulcers.

a one-day once-a-week fast

Taking 'time out' from food once a week is highly beneficial. In addition to giving your digestive system a rest, it naturally reduces your overall food intake.

To help you make this a part of your regular lifestyle, it is best to fast on the same day each week – you may like to choose a day when work is not too busy, or perhaps Monday as a recovery period after any excesses of the weekend.

It is important while fasting not to limit your intake of fluids. In addition to plain water, drink plenty of lime and honey water and fasting tea (see box, opposite). Unless you are able to make your fasting day a day of rest, you may need a little extra sustenance: you may eat fruit (but avoid citrus fruits, pineapples, mangoes and avocados) or make up a vegetable broth, using all sorts of vegetables except potatoes.

a three-day fast

This sort of fast can be done in a retreat or in the first few days of a holiday. It is a safe and very helpful fast that I recommend you do a couple of times a year, especially after Christmas or any other festive or over-indulgent period.

The basic principle is that you start off with no other food than liquid. The other two days include some basic, easily digestible foods so that there are no complications such as headaches, dizziness, fainting, hypoglycaemia or diarrhoea.

Although the release of toxins during fasting can cause some unpleasant side effects and moods or irritability, you should not be deterred, because the benefits are many. On average, people lose around 2 kg in the three days. This, of course, is mostly water, rather than fat, as fasting can reduce fluid retention, but it is encouraging and gives you a less bloated or puffy feeling.

organizing your fast

🍎 **The day before:** This is not a fast of complete abstinence, so ensure you have the following in stock (it is not a good idea to go out shopping while you are fasting):

- 🍎 2 limes
- 🍎 good organic honey
- 🍎 ingredients for fasting tea; teabags of relaxation tea (see below)
- 🍎 a selection of vegetables that can be eaten raw or lightly steamed
- 🍎 a selection of non-citrus fruits
- 🍎 ingredients for breakfast and supper on Day 3 (see pages 96–7).

It is also helpful to empty your fridge and cupboards of any tempting instant snacks.

Don't prepare for your fast by eating as much as possible 'to keep you going' – this is quite the wrong approach! Instead, wind down your digestion and prepare your body by having a light supper, perhaps vegetable soup and some fruit.

LIQUID SUSTENANCE

Lime and honey water: Fill a jug with 2 litres of water. Add 2 tbsp honey (warm so you can stir it into the water) and squeeze in the juice of half a lime (not more than this, as it would make the water too acidic).

Fasting tea: To 1½ litres of water add 2 cinnamon sticks, 6 cloves, 1 tbsp aniseed and 2 tbsp dried cranberries (optional). Boil for five minutes and leave to infuse.

Relaxation tea: Chamomile or other calming herbal teas.

Day 1: Prepare a large jug of lime and honey water (see box, page 95) and have a glass of this every 90 minutes or so throughout the day. Also drink three or four cups of fasting tea (see box, page 95) or chamomile tea without honey or sugar. You may also drink plain water whenever you want.

Have two showers a day, morning and evening. If you feel tired or sense the beginning of a headache, massage your neck and shoulders with a soothing massage oil. This will ease the fatigue and headache.

An alternative to massage is a relaxing bath. Fill the bath with warm water, not too hot. Add some soothing aromatic bath salts or oil, such as lavender. Soak your body and imagine that your muscles are relaxing and the blood vessels in them dilating. Do retention breathing: breathe in for three seconds, hold your breath for six seconds and breathe out slowly over six seconds. Remain in the bath for 10 minutes. Dry yourself and lie flat on your back for 10 minutes as you may feel light-headed.

Have an early night after a cup of relaxation tea – and ignore any dreams of delicious food or temptations you may have to get up and snack on chocolates or ice cream.

Day 2: Prepare the day's jug of lime and honey water, as yesterday, for drinking throughout the day.
Breakfast: bananas, apples, grapes, pears and melons, with fasting tea.
Lunch: a large bowl of non-citrus fruits.
Dinner: a plate of steamed vegetables: carrots, broccoli, peas, beans and baby corn and a bowl of salad (carrots, cucumber, radish, salad leaves).
Follow the same bathing, showering, massage and bedtime routine as Day 1.

Day 3: *Breakfast:* bowl of non-citrus fruits; cottage cheese with honey; 10 almonds, peeled and soaked for 24 hours; fasting tea.

KHICHRI RICE

Wash half a cup of basmati rice thoroughly. Put the rice and half a cup of lentils (soaked all day in plenty of cold water) into a large saucepan with 8 cups of water, a pinch of ground turmeric and a little salt and olive oil. Bring to simmering under a slow heat and cook until both rice and lentils are soft. Stir through to mix thoroughly.

Lunch: plate of salad (lettuce, carrots, cucumber, radish, spring onions with a dash of olive oil and lemon dressing) and a plate of cooked vegetables (potatoes, beans, broccoli, aubergines, peas, cauliflower), either stir fried or steamed.

Dinner: khichri rice (see above) with a little live yoghurt and steamed or stir-fried vegetables.

Follow the same bathing, showering, massage and bedtime routine as Day 1.

🍎 *Follow-up:* The fast is an effort, so do not ruin the benefits by immediately returning to a full diet, and especially do not eat a lot of heavy or junk food. Reintroduce your body to regular eating with a light vegetarian diet to stabilize the weight loss and then, day by day, introduce fish, eggs, chicken and meat in that order.

🍎 *Variations:* Those with the will-power and who are not afraid of fasting can do two days of liquid-only diet. If you have done the three-day fasts a few times, you can, in stages, prolong it up to seven days, as long as you are under the guidance of a qualified naturopath.

Do not venture on your own with a liquid-only fast beyond seven days, as you may get disconnected at times and lose control of your body, and the healing crisis (see page 99) could hit you. I wonder sometimes how hunger strikers handle the healing crisis – which they must go through if they are genuinely without food.

about long fasts

Conditions for which long, medically supervised fasting works well include obesity, osteoarthritis, manic depression, schizophrenia, eczema, psoriasis, chronic colitis, rheumatoid arthritis, allergies and food intolerances (except nut allergies), bronchial asthma, chronic bronchitis, sinusitis, mouth ulcers, migraine and chronic fatigue.

Ideally, fasting therapy is accompanied by massage, sauna or steam treatments, swimming or hydrotherapy, light exercise, meditation and art therapy (patients become very creative when undergoing long fasts). These treatments act synergistically with fasting to produce optimum results. Massage, meditation, light exercise and fasting in combination are a powerful form of therapy, arousing the innate healing power. In ancient Greece, all patients went through this combined therapy first as, in the majority of cases, that was all that was needed to kickstart the healing process. No medicine or other therapeutic interventions such as blood-letting were used unless the patient did not respond.

🍎 Before any medical fast, a thorough blood test is done to check for any abnormality or deficiency. Although the target number of fasting days is set, the actual duration of the fast depends on the condition of the patient, physically and mentally.

🍎 For the first two or three days, one feels very hungry. The thought of food dominates the day and at night there are dreams of delicious food. Hot baths, massages, sauna and lots of fluids help to eliminate the fatigue. This is when patients need maximum support as they are nervous, irritable and often scared. Some are very calm, as they know that it is a passing phase.

After three days, the hunger pangs miraculously stop. It is as if one does not want to eat. The body begins to feel lighter, the head clearer and sleep improves. One looks forward to bedtime as sound sleep lifts the mood. One feels great for another week. All symptoms of disease disappear.

Then, between the ninth and eleventh days, things take a turn for the worse again. This is the classic healing crisis. Everything gets worse – headaches, lethargy, palpitations, irritability and body aches. The original conditions for which the fast was recommended also get worse. The eczema, psoriasis, arthritic pain, swollen joints, migraine or whatever, which disappeared after the third day return with a vengeance. Itchy skin may be accompanied by a continuous headache. Patients panic because they have been symptom-free for a week. The healing crisis has been reached.

Until this point, patients have been encouraged to do light exercise, such as walking, swimming or yoga, but during the two days or so of healing crisis they are confined to bed. At this stage the physician conducting the fasting has to skilfully explain about the healing crisis: that things have to come out of the system, and that one has to feel worse before one is cured. During this period a lot of fluids are given. Light massages, enemas or colonic irrigation can help. Blood tests show bizarre results. The liver enzymes rise and kidney functions alter. Sometimes a drip is necessary. A small amount of glucose, given intravenously, keeps physiological symptoms at bay.

A couple of days later, like a miracle, things change again. The body calms down and all the symptoms of the original disease vanish. The

FAST AND SLOW

During a very long fast, the body conserves energy and the metabolism drops to the bare minimum, rather like an animal in hibernation, allowing the heart to beat, the lungs to breathe, and minimal movement, such as turning from side to side. When yogis go into controlled *samadhi*, they slow down their vital functions at will and go into a long trance lasting several days.

skin looks better, the eyes look clearer and moods return to normal. Light exercise is resumed.

🍎 After the healing crisis one has to wait for at least a week before fasting is discontinued. All the remnant symptoms of disease go away and the patient feels absolutely healthy. At this stage patients become very creative. Since no energy is lost in digestion, it is sublimated into creativity: typically, people compose poems, write about experiences, paint, sketch and even try their hands at chiselling or sculpting. This happens as if the mind and body is completely healed.

When obese people undertake a long fast like this, the weight loss gives them a great sense of motivation to continue the diet or fasting recommended by their physician. They feel light and elated, revelling in every word of praise and support from family and friends.

breaking the fast
Breaking the fast is a very important process. You do not want to undo the effort and sacrifice by eating rubbish or overloading your stomach, just as you would not feed a newborn baby something other than milk.

 The first three days of introduction of food after prolonged fasting are important. Patients start with runny rice soup or porridge only, two or three times a day. Normally, we numb our tastebuds by giving them too many complicated tastes at once. After fasting, the ability to taste becomes so accentuated that every morsel of food is blissful, and tastes heavenly. We should eat foods to stimulate one or two of the tastes at a time.

 After a day or two, vegetable soups are introduced, then steamed vegetables and only after four days salads or fruits (as they contain powerful enzymes). Next, some easily digested protein: soft-boiled eggs, the finest source of protein, and then low-fat chicken soup. The longer patients stay on a simple diet of fruit, vegetables, boiled rice, eggs, lentils and porridge, the better the system.

After long fasts, it is recommended that patients keep up a once-weekly fast (see page 94) for the rest of their life and about every three months take a two- or three-day fast, as described on page 94.

CAUTION

I must stress that fasts of more than a few days must be done under qualified supervision and closely controlled. Done correctly, longer fasting can have astonishing results, as Professor Nikolaev and his colleagues proved, and as traditional practices in India and elsewhere have shown. Fasting restores health and removes excess body fat and undesired deposits in blood vessels. It slows down the growth of cancers and may sporadically bring about remissions.

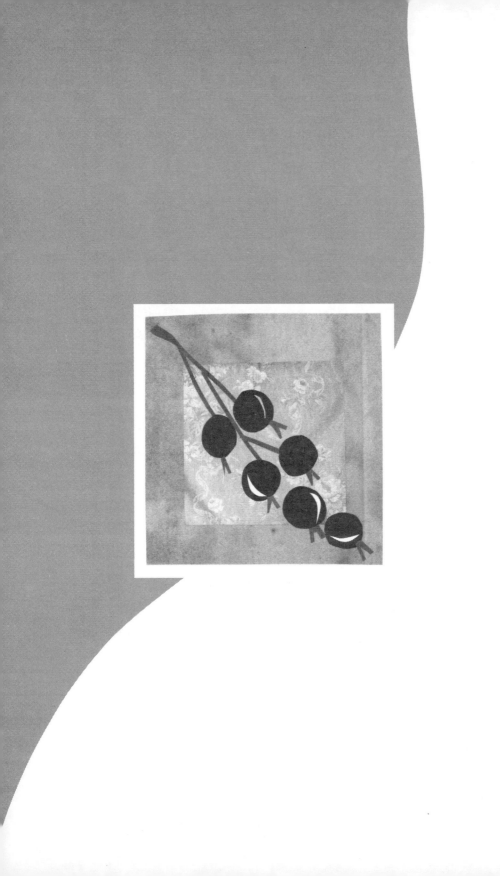

Regulating What You Eat

When and what and how much we eat can be triggered by several factors other than real hunger: a craving for a particular food, a 'false message' from the appetite centre or the stomach, a psychological desire to chew or eat, a tempting advertisement or smell, or just seeing other people enjoying food. We have seen in Chapter 4 how these different messages work on our eating habits, but here is some practical guidance on how to deal with them.

stomach acid

I view controlling stomach acidity as key to regulating appetite and weight gain. High stomach acid is the root cause of digestive problems, increased appetite and subsequent weight gain. But what can you do to avoid a build-up of stomach acidity?

avoid acidic fruit

This means not just citrus fruits such as oranges, grapefruits and lemons, but also:

- pineapple
- mango
- passion fruit
- kiwi fruit
- rhubarb
- gooseberries
- strawberries, raspberries, blackberries and their relations
- red-, black- and whitecurrants
- any sour varieties of fruit such as grapes and apples.

Many people are misled into thinking that the sharper the fruit, or the more 'bite' it has, the more vitamin C it contains – certain varieties of oranges have been bred to be so tart that you can feel their juice irritating your throat. While it is true that vitamin C (ascorbic acid) is best preserved in an acid medium (citric acid in the case of sour fruits), many other fruits and vegetables contain vitamin C in sufficient quantity to cater for daily needs and, frankly, scurvy is not a likely threat. In my opinion, the harm done to the stomach, digestion in general and possible weight gain due to increased appetite is of more concern.

Instead, get your vitamin C from:

- apples (sweet varieties)
- pears
- plums
- apricots
- peaches/nectarines
- papaya

BLACKCURRANTS

These are very rich in vitamin C, a powerful antioxidant that helps to strengthen the immune system, prevent heart disease and aid the body's struggle against infections, cancer and arthritis. Blackcurrants retain their vitamin C content better than many other sources, even when cooked or preserved. The professor under whom I studied in Moscow used to boil dried blackcurrants in water for patients on prolonged fasts (see page 91). He found the traditional lime and honey water too harsh for the fasting stomach, but blackcurrants provided vital vitamin C while keeping hunger pangs at bay.

- cherries
- figs
- dates
- tomatoes (in moderation, and choose large, sweet varieties – the outer flesh is less acidic than the inner pulp)
- leafy greens such as cabbage and salad leaves.

This is not to say that you must totally ban citrus and sour fruits from your diet, but don't think of them as the best source of vitamin C (weight for weight, lightly cooked Brussels sprouts provide more vitamin C than an orange). When you do choose citrus fruit remember that:

- sweet varieties such as satsumas or clementines are less acidic
- the whole fruit is better than just the juice as the fibres and pith, which are alkaline and bitter in taste, may help to neutralize the fruit's acid – an example of nature providing both acid and alkali in the same package.

Vitamin C is vulnerable to heat, so you will get most benefit by eating vegetables and fruit raw or only lightly cooked. Vitamin C is also water-

IS IT TRUE?

There is a commonly circulating myth that drinking lime or lemon juice in water first thing in the morning burns off fat. I don't know where it started, but the truth is that no one has ever lost weight this way – in fact, lemon and lime stimulate the appetite as they 'sharpen' the tastebuds.

soluble, so preserve as much vitamin C as possible by using minimal water, or by using the cooking water, for instance, as a base for soups or sauces.

minimize stomach irritants
Many foods can irritate the lining of the stomach, causing increased secretion of acid. Be particularly aware of:

Spicy food: Herbs and spices are very welcome for the extra flavour they bring to food when you are cutting out fat and salt to a large degree. Just don't overdo it, and see page 34 for the addictive nature of chillies.

The following herbs and spices are helpful to the digestion while adding flavour and interest to dishes:

- cumin
- ginger
- parsley
- coriander
- thyme
- spring onions
- rosemary.

Drugs: Some medicinal drugs (including many painkillers) are acidic in nature or irritate the digestive system. If you regularly need to take any drugs of this nature (your doctor or pharmacist, or an accompanying leaflet should identify acidic medication), avoid taking them on an empty stomach. You can alleviate the effects by taking them with a meal of at least something that will protect your stomach, such as porridge or milk.

Scalding hot food and drinks: An easy one to avoid.

Tea and coffee: Milk helps to neutralize the acid of black (Indian-style) tea. Chinese or Japanese green teas are less acidic, as are many herb teas, although strong spice teas, such as clove or cardamom, can be problematic.

Nuts, seeds, deep-fried food: Although the oils in fried foods, nuts and seeds create a feeling of satisfaction by coating the lining of the stomach and blocking the hunger receptors, their hardness or rough coatings encourage acidity as the stomach is faced with breaking them down. I advise avoiding deep-fried foods on any weight loss plan, and you can ease your stomach in processing nuts and other hard, rough foods by chewing every mouthful well.

A DELICIOUS DOUBLE WHAMMY

Nuts are highly calorific, and their smooth oiliness can become addictive. Chocolate is also high in calories and potentially addictive. Put the two together, and nutty chocolate is delivering a double whammy that spells danger to all efforts to lose weight.

other ways to regulate acidity

🍎 Eat slowly: allow your tastebuds to do their job (see page 32) and chew your food thoroughly to aid digestion.

🍎 Keep regular meal times: an empty stomach is an acidic stomach.

🍎 Avoid stress: a tense body needs more energy (food) and stress causes hypersecretion of stomach acid. Stress can also cause nervous overeating. Three good reasons to take up relaxing and de-stressing techniques (see Chapters 11 and 12).

🍎 Have regular neck massages: improving the flow of blood to the appetite centre in the hypothalamus will stop it sending messages for more glucose.

ALKALINE ALCOHOL ALERT

You may be surprised to discover that even alkaline alcoholic drinks, such as bitter aperitifs, beers, and spirits with angostura bitters, can increase stomach acidity. If the stomach receives a large amount of an alkaline substance, or has to cope with regular doses of alkalines, it secretes extra acid to counteract the effect, and sometimes overcompensates – which is why people who regularly take antacids often notice a 'rebound effect'.

yeasts

In addition to upsetting the balance of the digestive system, an excess of yeast in the gut can contribute to weight gain. Help control a proliferation of yeast by avoiding or minimizing how much you eat of:

🍎 bread (including pizza bases and many flat breads, such as pitta and naan, which contain yeast even though they do not rise)

🍎 beer

- yeast extract spreads
- soy sauce
- brewer's yeast (often used as a B vitamin supplement)
- many canned products.

craving and snacking

Cravings can be either physical or psychological, or a mixture of the two. It is possible for almost any food to become the focus of a craving, but avoiding those that can more easily lead to addiction is a sensible move, so minimize your intake of:

- sweet things, especially chocolate
- alcohol
- chillies.

Cravings, especially for something sweet, most usually come from demands from a brain that is sending messages that it needs glucose. This is particularly common mid-afternoon, when your energy is flagging, either because of the effort diverted to digesting lunch or because you have skipped lunch altogether.

To reduce the constant need to snack, and to dampen food cravings, instigate a regular mealtime regime and, unless you are following one of the more restrictive diets outlined on pages 155–66, use this simple guide to food combining.

- Breakfast: carbohydrates, to give a slow release of energy through the morning.
- Lunchtime: protein and vegetables.
- Evening: a lighter meal of carbohydrates and vegetables.

NIGHT-TIME MUNCHIES

If you return home late hungry and tired, don't make a full meal, but don't go to bed hungry – either way you will have a disturbed sleep. Instead, make a soothing drink, such as chamomile or peppermint tea with a little honey, and have one or two plain biscuits.

Midnight snacking, or eating heavy meals late at night, is a major cause of weight gain. If you stay up late, four or five hours after dinner, you will feel hungry again, even at night (insomniacs often get an attack of the munchies). Going to bed two or three hours after dinner is ideal; your digestion will then be well underway.

If your evening meal has to be your main meal of the day, you will probably need to eat your protein then, but try not to eat too late. And do not go all day without eating – lunch is an important meal in the battle against cravings.

If you still feel the need to snack, opt for fruit, not sweets or sandwiches.

planning meals

You feel hungry mid-morning and raid the fridge or biscuit tin for 'a little something to keep you going ...' You have missed lunch and feel a desperate need mid-afternoon to dash to the corner shop where the only choice is a fatty pasty or bars of chocolate ... There's nothing for supper so you ring for a takeaway ... Losing weight is much harder if you do not plan ahead.

Once a week, sit down and plan all the week's meals. If you are not the one who does the shopping or cooking, you will need to do this together, and you will need to plan meals for the whole family. This may entail a whole new way of thinking and at first it may seem time-consuming, but in the longer term it can save you time and money as well as weight.

shopping

Like so many other food-related things, shopping is often a matter of habit. We are inclined to follow the same routine week after week. Look afresh at how, when and where you get your food, and you may find that you can make small changes that make a big difference.

Make a shopping list. This sounds obvious, but sticking to a list may be easier said than done, because supermarkets in particular are adept at subliminal 'Buy me' messages: sweets by the check-out where you cannot rush by; pots of cream enticingly placed next to punnets of strawberries; hard-to-resist multi-buy special offers.

The list should cover at least a week, but how often you shop depends on your lifestyle and other commitments. You will need to balance the temptation that food shopping inevitably carries, with the advantage of buying and eating food as fresh as possible.

Your list should include quantities as well as specific items. Buying too much food will either result in wastage or, because we hate to see food

---

IS SHOPPING ONLINE THE ANSWER?

Shopping online may be helpful, but you will not be able to choose your own fresh food. Depending on the shopping facilities available to you, a satisfactory answer may be to buy grocery basics online and then bypass the enticements of the supermarket shelves by buying fresh food from specific shops: butchers, greengrocers, etc. You are much less likely to succumb to impulse buying or over-buying if you have to ask for each item individually.

go to waste, eating up the excess to stop it spoiling. Buying too little, on the other hand, will just mean turning to the quick fix of a pre-prepared supermarket meal, a takeaway or eating out before the week is over.

preparing and cooking

Cook just enough food for the meal, so that there are no leftovers to snack on. An exception to this is if you are specifically planning to use them for a meal the next day – for instance, extra rice to make a rice salad. If you are used to cooking for a family you may not have adjusted to buying and cooking smaller amounts of food once the children have left home.

Being the only one in a family following a strict weight-loss diet can be particularly difficult, so you will need to find ways that work for everyone. The rest of the family may not wish to cut out all fats, for instance, but at least a temporary ban on sweets, cakes and biscuits would be a healthy move for the whole family and provide fewer tempting snacks for you.

Regulating your eating habits is much easier if you only have yourself to cater for, but family eating patterns are inevitably influenced by all members of the family. Even if you have not discerned a genetic aspect to your weight problem from your self-assessment (see page 78), you

SUGAR AND FAT SUBSTITUTES

Sugar substitutes such as aspartame, as used in 'diet' colas, 'sugar-free' desserts and in tea or coffee, help to reduce the need for consumption of sugar by fooling the tastebuds. Fat substitutes used in the food industry do a similar job, convincing the tastebuds that they are identifying the rich smoothness of cream and butter even though they are not. These substitutes are in reality catering for the emotional needs that food provides rather than fulfilling the body's true demand for glucose or fats.

may find it extremely useful to read Chapter 15, which includes many tips on how to incorporate healthy eating into family life.

when socializing ...

Whether it's a celebratory party, a business lunch or a relaxed dinner with friends, we all know that social occasions are when we are most likely to over-indulge. In fact, the advice for regulating what you eat at these times is no different from any other – it's just that it's easier to lose track because you are probably paying attention to the conversation or entertainment rather than to the food. Being presented with an array of delicious food, and quite possibly an awful lot of it, also makes it harder to keep to a sensible regime.

On pages 167–9 are more specific guidelines for eating out when you are following a strict diet, but the following are helpful at any time to guard against over-eating.

Eat slowly: Trying to participate in a discussion while eating encourages you to gulp your food. Because you want to empty your mouth as quickly as possible, you don't savour the food, you don't chew properly and you swallow air as you hurriedly dispatch another mouthful.

If you have a choice of food, choose dishes that will help you to eat more slowly:

🍎 soup will force you to pause as you concentrate on not spilling the spoonful; it is also easy to digest

🍎 food that needs thorough chewing draws your attention to what you are eating and keeps you alert

🍎 fish or meat that needs to be cut off the bone requires more concentration than filleted or diced cuts

🍎 vegetables such as asparagus or broccoli need more attention than peas or purées.

Get into a rhythm of chew and listen, stop and talk. Give the other person a chance to do the same. Set a calm pace (and remember that there is a lot to be said for listening more than you talk).

Make a conscious choice of food: Remind yourself beforehand to guard against saying Yes for the sake of appearances or to please your host/guest.

Choose from a menu or a buffet with your head, not your eyes. Look for dishes that will provide a satisfying meal while intruding as little as possible into your 'Avoid' list.

If helpings are large, do not feel obliged to eat everything on your plate; despite the distractions, pay attention to what your body is telling you.

Choose only a very light dessert or none at all – you are unlikely still to be hungry.

Keep count of the drinks: This can be the toughest part of a social occasion, especially if you do not have to drive home afterwards. Often, people will say they'll just have a couple of drinks early in the evening and then switch to soft drinks. The trouble is that even quite a small amount of alcohol on an empty stomach, especially an acidic drink such as white wine, stimulates the appetite, so you are actually preparing the ground for eating more than you intend.

Have a soft drink before the meal and enjoy a glass of wine at the table. Taking the wine in sips with food will slow down the absorption time of the alcohol (and sipping it will also give you more pleasure). If you are entertaining or being entertained regularly you may find it preferable to avoid alcoholic drinks altogether – socially an increasingly acceptable option.

Mitigate the effects: If, despite your vigilance, you know you have eaten too much, keep meals for the next couple of days very simple; a one-day full fast (see page 94) will help redress the balance.

CASE STUDY

When I first saw Debbie she was aged about 40, weighed 110 kg, suffered from recurrent heartburn and headaches, chronic fatigue and her periods had become irregular. She had tried several diets but these only sapped her strength further and did nothing for her craving for sweet things. She worried all the time about her weight and health and was on prescribed antidepressants. I discovered that she had had a car accident in her twenties, from which she had suffered whiplash injuries, and that her weight problems began a few years after that.

I put her on a regime of three-day fasts and a once-a-week fast. She received neck massage weekly and was given kadu tea for her candida and to help control her sugar cravings. These measures regulated her stomach acidity, appetite, cravings and water retention. They also increased her energy so that she was able to go for a swim or walk regularly.

In six months, she lost almost 20 kg on just the treatments given, with no extra-restrictive diet, and looked extremely well.

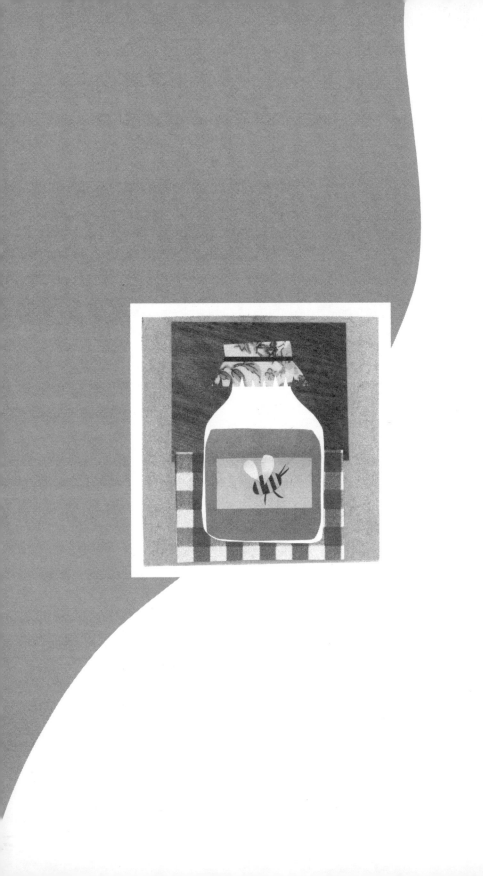

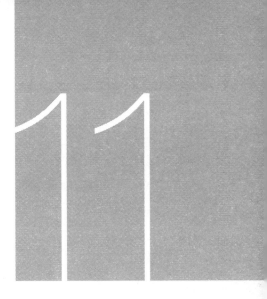

Therapeutic Yoga and Exercise

It is common sense that exercise helps you lose weight, as it draws on the fat your body is storing. Exercise done alongside a controlled weight loss plan has a greater impact than either one on their own.

Many forms of exercising are useful to regulate excess body weight. If you are not used to exercising, it is important to begin slowly and build up, taking professional guidance where necessary (for instance, in a gym). It is also important to keep up a regular regime – throwing yourself into a session at the gym or a long run to the point of exhaustion and then doing nothing for another month will have no beneficial effect at all.

where to start?

If you are very overweight you should begin very gently. Talk to your doctor, and plan together a programme suited to your weight and fitness.

You may well not be able to bend or stretch easily, but that will change as you lose some weight and your body becomes stronger and more supple. The following are all good starting points:

Walking. An excellent form of all-round exercise at any level. If even a daily walk in the park is more than you are used to, begin with this. Walk purposefully, swinging your arms, rather than just wandering, and set yourself increasing targets, both in time and distance. What you do at the beginning will probably not be invigorating power-walking, but it will still improve your breathing and your arm and leg muscles. It will also use up stored energy, i.e. fat.

Swimming. This is another really good form of exercise, especially if you are very overweight, as it takes all strain off your joints. In the water you can feel as light as a supermodel! Don't feel embarrassed about appearing in public half-naked: most pools have sessions specifically for adults or 'seniors', and if you haven't been to a pool for years you may be surprised at the variety of sizes and shapes of the swimmers. If you can't swim, you will probably find that there are lessons with a group of like-minded (and like-shaped) people.

Exercises for the arms, back and legs are geared to all levels of ability. A regular class is good for motivation or morale, but you can also do these at home. Books, videos and TV programmes are all sources of suitable stretches and movements, and your local surgery or clinic may have hand-out sheets of recommended exercises tailored to the overweight. Incorporating light hand-held or strap-on weights (2–3 kg) will make your muscles work harder on even simple movements.

Dance. Dancing may only seem like a bit of fun, but all forms, including stately ballroom dancing, provide good aerobic exercise as well as improving posture and coordination. Music is a good aid to relaxation, and moving to music provides a pleasurable antidote to the stresses and strains of life.

Yoga. I list this last, but it is one of the very best forms of exercise and one suited to all weights, shapes and ages. The controlled breathing calms the mind, and the *asanas* (poses) invigorate and work the body without strain. Done regularly, yoga relieves stress and the good posture and relaxation techniques help keep the pituitary well controlled, reducing hormonal problems. Because of its multiple benefits, it is on yoga that I want to focus the rest of this chapter. I believe that if the principles of yoga were to be followed by everyone, weight gain would cease to be a problem unless there were some genetic or constitutional background.

yoga for everyone

Different yoga *asanas* (poses) can help to act on specific areas of fat on the abdomen, thighs, trunk, neck and arms. Even though most of the *asanas* tend to look very slow, their effect is powerful. Some of the balancing poses and those involving anti-gravitational forces – such as the Swan (balancing the body horizontally on two hands) or the Half Peacock (handstand) are extremely strenuous exercises as the muscles are put to test with the body's own weight.

Vigorous versions of yoga such as asthanga yoga are becoming increasingly popular. Bikram Chowdhury's 'hot yoga' (doing yoga at 40°C) makes you sweat as if you have done a marathon and the heat helps to remove stiffness in the body and enables you to get into postures that you normally could not. However, yoga does not have to

YOGA PRINCIPLES

Yoga goes far beyond the basic poses and stretches practised in a typical yoga class. It is a complete, integrated system that gives you a balanced lifestyle. Here are some yogic principles that help with weight loss.

 Foods should be fresh and natural. We are surrounded nowadays by conveniently packaged, pre-prepared food with long shelf-lives, mass-produced for cheapness. These are unlikely to conform to yogic principles of freshness and naturalness.

 Food is consumed to provide nourishment to the body and mind. It can be classified into three categories:

Sattvic: healthy foods to increase energy and vitality, contributing to a balanced diet of less fat, sufficient protein and only essential amounts of carbohydrate

Rajasic: foods that excite the body's functions and rely heavily on the tastes, categorized as bitter, sour, pungent, astringent, salty and sweet

Tamasic: foods that are putrid and rotten, and cause illness. Today's preserved foods, while not decomposed, fall into this category and can cause digestive problems.

 No excess consumption of food.

 Fasting or only eating fruits on special days of the year, including the first day of total darkness (new moon).

 Eat three meals a day and the last should be eaten at dusk. Never eat late.

 Rest after lunch.

 Eat when you are hungry.

 Do Bajrasana or the Thunderbolt pose after eating a meal (see page 45).

 Yoga exercises, done in a sequence with correct breathing, act as fat-burners.

be done like this to be effective. Whether you choose to do a sequence of slow but intense postures or fast and vigorous ones is your own choice. Ultimately, both will lead you to similar results.

Yoga does not require any props or special clothes, so it can be done in the comfort of your own home and in your own time. Incorporating 30 minutes of yoga into your daily routine helps it become a regular part of your life, and during a weight loss programme it is an excellent way to start the morning, a form of ritual that allows you to begin each day in an optimistic frame of mind.

One of the greatest advantages of yoga is that it harmonizes the body and the mind. Digestion, blood pressure, hormonal balance, weight and general well-being all automatically improve as your body's various forces regulate themselves.

Included here are some of the poses that are particularly helpful in a weight loss programme.

the art of breathing

Pranayama or breathing is perhaps the most scientific aspect of yoga. The haemoglobin in red blood cells exchanges carbon dioxide for oxygen, molecule for molecule. Retention breathing, as practised in yoga, tends to build up carbon dioxide levels in the blood, which is exchanged for oxygen in the lungs. So, the more slowly you breathe, the more oxygenated the blood becomes. Increased oxygen coupled with the controlled body movements of the *asanas* helps to burn stored energy, first the sugar and, ultimately, fat deposits.

Breathing exercises need some practice and guidance. Normally most people draw in their abdomen when breathing in, expanding the chest above. This is incorrect. Relaxing the abdomen helps the diaphragm to flatten out and allows the lungs room to inhale the maximum amount of air.

Ujjayi (abdominal breathing): Sit comfortably in the lotus pose or on a chair. Close your mouth. Inhale slowly through both nostrils, allowing your abdomen to relax and your chest to expand. Picture your lungs filling up with air. Hold your breath for as long as you comfortably can (20 seconds or so). Then slowly breathe out. Draw the abdomen in and let the chest collapse to original position. This will allow your diaphragm to return to its dome shape as it is lifted up and the result will be total exhalation. Repeat this 10 times. Both this and the next breathing exercise generate heat in the body.

Bhastrika (complete breath): This is similar to *Ujjayi* but done more rapidly. Using the same technique, inhale and exhale rapidly in quick succession 15–20 times (fewer if you feel dizzy or light-headed). Then hold your breath for 20 seconds, and repeat the rapid breathing 15–20 times. Repeat this sequence 5–10 times.

Kapala Bhati (forceful exhalation): This clears the head and generates heat in the body. Do not do this if you have high blood pressure, a hernia, an ulcer, prolapsed organs in the lower abdomen or suffer from eye or ear complaints.

Inhale and quickly exhale forcefully. To give the right amount of force, pull your abdomen right in as you exhale. As you do this, the diaphragm is pushed up and the chest is drawn in, expelling the maximum air. As the muscles relax the air is automatically drawn into the lungs without conscious inhalation. The abdomen does not bellow out as that would delay the whole process – the emphasis is on forcing the air out: 'whoosh … whoosh'. The quicker you exhale the better. Do 15–20 exhalations, hold your breath for 15–20 seconds and repeat the cycle 5–10 times.

Sukh Purvak (alternate nostril breathing): This calms the mind and relaxes the body. Close your right nostril with your right thumb, inhale slowly through the left nostril. Fill your lungs to full capacity, using your abdomen and chest as before. Now, close the left nostril with a finger and exhale slowly through the right nostril, drawing the abdomen in and relaxing the chest. Now do the same in reverse, inhaling through the right nostril and exhaling through the left nostril. Repeat this slow rhythmic breathing cycle 15–20 times.

yoga poses

After completing this set of breathing exercises, move on to the physical *asanas*, or yogic postures. The following two *asanas* improve blood flow into the head, irrigating the pituitary gland and helping hormonal balance.

Setubandhasana (semi-bridge or shoulder pose): Lie on your back with your arms by your side, palms down. Bend both legs at the knees, keeping your heels hip-distance apart. Take a deep breath in and lift your pelvis as high as you can. Draw down your chin to touch your upper chest. Continue to hold your breath in this pose for a few seconds. You will feel the blood rushing to your head, eyes, face and neck. Lower your hips to the floor slowly as you breathe out, keeping your knees the same distance apart the whole time. Bring your chin back to the original position. Repeat 5 times.

Pawan Mukt (wind-relieving pose): This posture relieves wind and constipation, reducing abdominal distension. It helps keeps the waist size in check, reducing bloating that may give the impression of fatness. A useful morning exercise.

Lie on your back with your legs stretched out and your arms by your side. Take a deep breath in and bring your right knee up towards your chest and hold it with your left hand, drawing your knee and thigh into your abdomen as you exhale. Bring your head up to touch your knee with the tip of your nose or chin. Hold for five seconds, then lower your head, release and extend your leg, breathing in as you do so. Repeat with the left leg. Repeat five times with each leg.

If you have difficulty achieving this position, it is still beneficial to hold the knee and press it against the abdomen, without lifting your head.

Surya Namaskar (salutation to the sun)

Surya Namaskar exercises all parts of the body, tuning them into harmony. It is an ideal cycle of postures to do each morning, to prepare for the day ahead. If you are very overweight, incorporate the salutation only when you have lost some weight, or it may strain your joints.

Once you can manage it, this sequence of *asanas* brings many benefits, and if done briskly really makes you sweat and burn off the fat. The stretching and compressing of muscles by this exercise helps eradicate obesity and makes the spine strong and flexible, improving the functions of the nervous system, the circulatory system and the hormonal system. It also brings flexibility to the joints and helps to create a sense of well-being through improved energy levels.

Move through each posture slowly, coordinating *Ujjayi*-style breathing to your movements. Ideally the sequence of twelve *asanas* should be done as one continuous, free-flowing movement. However, this might be possible only after some practice.

1. *Namaskar Asana:* Stand erect, feet together or a little apart, with hands held palms together in front of your chest, in an attitude of prayer. Your weight should be properly balanced on your feet. Relax, and concentrate on your breathing. This will calm your mind.

2. *Urdh Namaskar Asana:* Inhaling, raise your arms above your head and bend backwards slightly. Hold this posture for a few seconds. It gives a backward stretch to the spine and activates the lungs fully.

3. *Hastpad Asana:* Exhaling, bend forwards, keeping the knees straight. Then bring your arms down and try to place the palms of your hands on the ground in line with your feet. Bring your forehead as close to your knees as you can. This stretches the spine and increases its flexibility. The lower part of the lungs and abdomen get compressed, exercising the abdominal organs. It reduces the waist, improves digestion and the bowel movement.

4. *Ekpad Prasar Asana:* Inhaling, take a big backward step with the right leg. Gradually touch the ground with your right knee and bend the left leg. Keep your hands on the ground and raise your head backwards. In this position the left thigh exerts a light pressure on the spleen, activating it. The neck is also exercised in this posture.

5. *Bhudar Asana:* Exhaling, take the left leg back too. Lift the right knee off the ground so that both legs are straight. Try to touch your heels on the ground and bring your head down while lifting your hips as much as you can, to form an inverted V shape with your body. Stretching and compressing of muscles melts away the fat. This also makes the ankles become very supple.

6. *Ashtang Paripat Asana*: Inhaling, bend both arms, lower your body to the floor so that knees, chest and forehead touch the ground, but keep your hips and abdomen as high as possible off the floor. The whole weight of the body is on the hands and the toes. Done regularly this squeezes off every fraction of useless fat, leaving the muscles clean and supple. Bending your head upwards (as if you were trying to see the ceiling) exercises the muscles of the neck and throat, preventing sagging and loosening of the skin. As so much of the body is supported by the hands, the wrists and the forearms, these joints get strengthened.

7. *Bhujang Asana:* Lower your hips to the floor and raise the upper part of your body on your arms, bending backwards to extend the spine as much as possible. As the whole weight is carried by the arms, they gradually become shapely, strong and supple. This makes the chest wider and deeper and improves the firmness and elasticity of the bust. Any tendency towards tonsillitis and other throat troubles is checked by this *asana*. The spine is also stretched and becomes more flexible.

8. Repeat Bhudar Asana, exercise 5.

9. Repeat Ekpad Prasar Asana, exercise 4, but this time bend the right leg and take your left leg backwards. The pressure exerted by the right thigh on the abdomen activates the liver.

10. Repeat Hastpad Asana, exercise 3.

11. Repeat Urdh Namaskar Asana, exercise 2.

12. Repeat Namaskar Asana, exercise 1.

If you practise this exercise sequence five to 10 times, five times a week, you will develop muscular strength and your endurance level will improve. It will increase the flexibility of your spine and limbs and improve your digestion and breathing capacity. Fat around the abdomen will be reduced and the body will become more shapely. It will also add grace and attractiveness to your movements and will help you to maintain youthful buoyancy.

ADVANCED SALUTATION TO THE SUN

To achieve the fullest benefits of Surya Namaskar, in addition to proper breathing, you should recite a specific mantra while concentrating on a designated point of the body. These points, known as plexuses, are centres of particularly powerful energy or concentrations of nerves and equate to yogic chakras. The posture, the area on which to concentrate and the mantra to be recited with its English version is given below:

	Asana	**Chakra**	**Mantra**	**English version**
1	Namaskar	Crown (top of head)	Om Mitraya Namah	Friend of all I bow to thee
2	Urdh Namaskar	Throat	Om Ravaye Namah	Praised by all I bow to thee
3	Hastpad	Navel (solar plexus)	Om Suryay Namah	Guide of all I bow to thee
4	Ekpad Prasar	Spleen	Om Bhanave Namah	Bestower of beauty I bow to thee
5	Bhudar	Third eye (between eyebrows)	Om Khagaya Namah	Stimulator of the senses I bow to thee
6	Ashtang Paripat	Heart	Om Pushne Namah	Nourisher of life I bow to thee
7	Bhujang	Base (perineum)	Om Hirangarbhaya Namah	Promoter of virility I bow to thee
8	Bhudar	Third eye (between eyebrows)	Om Marichaye Namah	Destroyer of disease I bow to thee
9	Ekpad Prasar	Spleen	Om Adityaya Namah	Inspirer of love I bow to thee
10	Hastpad	Navel (solar plexus)	Om Savitre Namah	Begetter of life I bow to thee
11	Urdh Namaskar	Throat	Om Arkaya Namah	Inspirer of awe I bow to thee
12	Namaskar	Crown (top of head)	Om Bhaskaraya Namah	Refulgent One I bow to thee

To finish your yoga session, go into the Corpse Pose:

 Shavasana (corpse pose): This may sound simple, but in fact it is the hardest posture to achieve because it is difficult to let your muscles relax as if you were in a deep sleep while remaining conscious. You will also gently stretch the back and sides of the neck and the shoulders, which helps to relax the whole body.

Lie on your back with your feet apart and your legs relaxing outwards. Keep your arms a little away from your trunk, palms facing up. Take a deep breath in and lower your chin to stretch the back of your neck away from your shoulders. Breathe out slowly to release the neck and shoulders, allowing them to 'sink' towards the floor. Relax your facial muscles. Check your breathing: your abdomen should rise on inhaling and fall on exhaling.

Take another deep breath in, lift your arms up and stretch them out on the ground behind your head. Flex your toes to stretch the back of your legs. Breathe out slowly and relax your arms, feet, legs and neck. Return to normal breathing and slowly lower your arms to your sides again.

Take a deep breath in and press your shoulders down, away from your neck. Stretch your fingers out and point to your toes with your outstretched arms. Breathe out slowly and relax again. Return to normal breathing.

Breathe in and turn your head to the right so that your right ear is touching the floor. Keep your left shoulder pressed down to the floor. Breathe out and keep this stretch. Then return to normal breathing. Relax the left side of your neck and shoulders. Stay like this for 2–3 minutes, relaxing your facial muscles, particularly in the jaw, by taking your tongue away from the roof of your mouth. Repeat on the other side.

Lie still and let your mind wander over your body, starting with your toes. Keep your breathing below the ribcage; it should be rhythmic, smooth and light, without any constrictions. Relax your muscles completely. Try to let the base of your skull sink deeper and deeper towards the floor. Check your breathing again. Stay in this posture for 20 minutes.

Slowly turn to the right with your right hand under your head. Relax, then slowly roll over and repeat on the left. Turn to the right again to stand up slowly.

The corpse pose is an excellent relaxation pose at the end of the day. It lowers your body temperature as you go into a state of relaxation, so make sure you are comfortably clothed, or you might feel cold.

My colleague Jiwan Brar and I wrote a book, *Therapeutic Yoga*, which explores the subject in much greater detail and includes some interesting explanations on the principles of therapeutic yoga. Perhaps it will convince you to use this as a preferential form of exercise of the mind and body. The Weight Loss DVD (see page 208) also demonstrates the various *asanas* described here.

Massage

You may already know it as a pleasant relaxant, but massage plays an active role in improving the way our bodies function, working on our muscles, our senses and our brains. It is also an invaluable part of any weight loss plan.

restoring energy

If muscles become stiff due to overproduction of lactic acid or from physical strain or injury, they fail to function as well as they should. A deep massage improves the blood flow to the muscles, invigorates them and makes them capable of producing energy once more.

When muscles go into spasm from fatigue, they present resistance to the millions of tiny capillaries in their tissues. The effect is a sluggish circulation, which causes overall lethargy as oxygen and nutrient supplies to various parts of the body, particularly the brain, are affected. Relieving this spasm is very useful for re-energizing the body.

Different massage techniques can also have specific effects.

Scratching the skin gently with the nails, slapping or pummelling, usually stimulates or makes the body more alert, whereas stroking, caressing and gentle squeezing has a relaxing effect.

massage as therapy

Massage is not only a pleasurable thing, but is also therapeutic. Massaging tendons or ligaments improves blood flow to them and if they are inflamed this will help them mend. Pressing sore areas sends messages to the brain and draws its attention to the affected area so that the healing powers of the body can focus on them.

Touch in itself is healing. The pleasant sensation achieved after a good session of therapeutic massage is in itself good for the mind and the body, and contributes to the healing or the adjustment towards a harmonious balance.

In my quest for identifying therapies that bring maximum benefit, I believe that massage is the most efficacious of them all. As explained in Chapter 6, I have found that healing takes place at the level of the sub-conscious brain, and that this part of the brain receives its blood supply through the vertebral arteries located inside the cervical (or neck) vertebrae. Massaging the neck area improves blood supply to vital parts of the brain that control functions as varied as the immune system, hormones, appetite

EMOTIONAL RESPONSES

The skin is full of receptors, which relate to various types of emotions. Stroking the nerve receptors under the arm, on the neck or on the soles of the feet, for instance, can make us giggle or laugh. The receptors on the scalp and the heels can induce sleep. There are erogenous receptors behind the ears, in the groin, on the inner thighs, the lower abdomen, lips, breasts, etc.

MEDICINAL MASSAGE

The therapeutic effects of massage were well understood by the ancient Greeks and Romans, whose baths and healing temples had skilled masseurs. Here people did not only get their physical aches and pains relieved but were also healed.

In India, China and other places, massage is used as a powerful form of treatment. Ayuvedic *panchkarma*, for example, uses medicated oils applied with a variety of strokes to impregnate the skin, so that the ingredients in the oils can enter the bloodstream, producing therapeutic effects. Conventional medicine also uses skin absorption – HRT patches work on this basis, for example. Administering medication in this way bypasses the liver, which often neutralizes or destroys many medicines taken orally.

and the digestive system as well as respiration, temperature control, sexual function, gait, posture and reproduction. I reached the logical conclusion that optimizing the blood flow to these nerve or control centres rectifies damage in the body and leads to healing and well-being. Time after time my success in treating ailments with neck and shoulder massage, yoga and gentle manipulation has proved my hypothesis correct.

therapeutic neck massage

As part of a weight loss plan, this neck and shoulder massage helps to improve pituitary–hypothalamic functions (see page 25). The effect of this is to reduce cravings and improve thyroid functions. It can also help to eradicate fluid retention.

This massage sequence is a great reliever of tension. This release of tension will make you feel very relaxed and, with the blood and the cerebrospinal fluid circulation to the brain increased, energized by a feel-good factor.

You cannot do this massage on yourself, so these instructions are for a friend or partner to massage you. Prepare yourself by lying face down, with a pillow under your neck and chest. Make sure you are comfortable and that your neck is relaxed and you can still breathe easily (it may help to support your forehead and chin on a rolled towel).

If you have had an injury or operation to the neck, suffer from osteoporosis, disc prolapse or have other problems with this area, massage should only be undertaken by a suitably qualified professional who is aware of your medical history in this respect.

🍎 Use a massage oil to maximize the effect of the massage (see box, page 137).

🍎 Place the four fingers of one hand on one side of the neck and your thumb on the other side, just below the ear lobes. (If you can't reach, you may use the fingers of both hands instead.) You should feel some bony projections on the sides of the neck. These are the sides of the cervical vertebrae that have deep within them the canal through which the vertebral arteries run. Sometimes these can be difficult to feel at first – severe muscle tension or a lot of fatty tissue makes them harder to locate – but you should find them if you use sufficient pressure.

🍎 Start massaging these protrusions in a rotatory fashion, and step down one vertebra at a time until you reach the last one above the shoulder. One or two protrusions may feel sore; these are the ones that have got out of alignment. Usually, it is the third cervical vertebra which is misaligned either to the left or right. Massage for five minutes or so, paying particular attention to these sore areas.

🍎 Next, keep your fingers on one side of the neck and your thumb on the other, but position them a little further in (by 2 cm or so) towards the central axis. Now you will feel cords of muscles. Massage these from the skull downwards. Some muscles will be sore. Start massaging them gently at first, and after a few strokes increase the pressure.

After a few minutes, position your fingers further inwards again. You will find some more muscles here. Massage them in the same way.

Then massage the nape of the neck, pinching with the thumb and the four fingers.

Next, massage the area of the occiput (the back of the skull), where the muscles of the neck are attached. This is usually above the hairline. You will feel that these are strong tendons and they can be very sore, especially when the neck muscles are tensed.

After doing this for a few minutes, take a firm hold on the muscles on top of the shoulder. Work on one shoulder at a time and use both hands to grasp the band of muscle, with your thumb on top and your fingers underneath. Massage both shoulders thoroughly, squeezing and kneading them. These are the trapezius muscles and are often very sore.

Finally, use your thumb and fingers to massage the jaw muscles on either side. Finish by massaging the jaw line and the temples as well.

The massage technique is demonstrated in more detail on my Lifestyle DVD (see page 208).

treating specific areas

As we have seen in Chapter 2, the body builds up deposits of white fat (cellulite) in specific areas of the body where it serves no useful function, forming insulation or cushioning, and does not interfere with the working of the body. This fat does not respond as well to diet or exercises as yellow fat, which derives from what we eat. Massage, surgery and liposuction become the only option for getting rid of cellulite. I do not recommend the latter two unless obesity is such that walking becomes almost impossible, there is a threat to the joints, and so on. Even then, diet, exercise and massage, as well as real motivation, have to come first or the fat that is removed will soon be replaced.

The areas that respond best to treatment are where cellulite tends to amass: the sides of the thighs, the upper arms, below the navel and across the lower abdomen, around the hips and over the buttocks, and on the breasts.

If you have cellulite deposits in several areas, treat just one or two at a time, so that you can give each a period of concentrated attention. The following day, move on to another area as the original one will be sore, and work round the affected areas of your body in a cycle, massaging each area in turn. If you have only one area that needs treating, allow a gap of a couple of days between massage sessions, more if you need it.

massaging away cellulite

This is a very vigorous form of massage. Remember you are trying to break up fat, so it will necessarily involve some pain and bruising later. Any technique that breaks up fat mechanically is likely to bruise, but this is only tissue bruising and should not cause concern.

Do not treat any areas that are affected by thread veins or varicose veins – or vulnerable areas around recent scar tissue or open sores.

 Apply massage oil to your hands, rub your palms together to warm it up and potentize (energize) it.

MASSAGE OILS

Any pleasant oil, such as almond, will facilitate massaging, but an oil specifically formulated for treating cellulite has added benefits. These oils contain ingredients such as mustard and ginger oils, which have a heating effect that is quite noticeable. This draws blood to the tissue being massaged and so improves the potency of the treatment. I have found that the synergistic effect of two high-quality oils, kalonji (black cumin) and mustard, to be a particularly powerful combination and this is what I use in my cellulite oil (see page 207), along with other ingredients such as ginger oil and saffron.

Because of the sometimes quite intense warming effect of cellulite oils, it is better not to treat yourself last thing at night, just before going to bed.

Not all the oil will be absorbed. Half an hour or so after massaging, wipe away the excess oil with surgical spirit, which will also assist in removing grease and moisture from the cellulite deposits, helping to reduce their mass. (Wear gloves for this, or the spirit will remove moisture from your fingers as well.)

Rub the oil into the area you are working on until it is fully absorbed by the skin. After that, knead the area by pinching and lifting the fat and skin folds between the thumbs and four fingers. Continue this for about five minutes. Do it gently at first and then apply more pressure as you get used to it.

It is beneficial to put hot towels on the area that you have worked on. Leave them in place for five minutes or so. This helps the absorbed oil to work better. After kneading the skin, you can warm up the tissue with friction, by rubbing the area briskly with the palm of your hand.

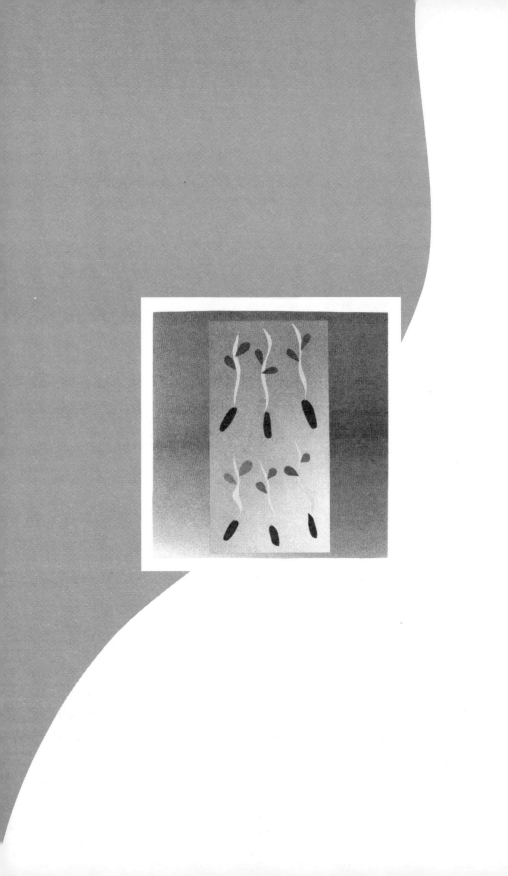

If You Eat Too Much and Exercise Too Little

If what you have read and learned so far has brought you to this chapter, you will have deduced that, for you, a successful weight loss plan is one that will bring back into balance the amount of energy that you take in (i.e. what you eat) and the amount that you use up. And that to lose weight you will have to take in less than you expend.

Before you begin a weight loss diet, you must set out a target weight. Use the body mass index chart on page 87 to help ascertain your optimum weight, and be realistic about how long it will take you to achieve it. Weight lost slowly and steadily will stay off much more effectively than a sudden drop.

It is probable that your weight loss will follow a typical pattern:

 an initial marked loss, which is very encouraging, but mostly due to reduced fluid retention and not loss of fat

 a slower loss of around 1 kg or 2 lb per week. Even if the weight loss is frustratingly slow, stay with the diet and exercise regime for at least 12 weeks

 a 'sticking point' – if, despite your best efforts, your weight stays the same over a two-week period, then that should indicate that you have reached a plateau. At this point, increase your exercise regime; normally this will result in further weight loss as your body's metabolic rate increases

 a second plateau – you should now have reached the maximum potential for this weight loss plan.

The plan I advise is:

 to follow the weight loss plan recommended here until you reach the first plateau.

 then continue with the same diet, but switch over to an intensive exercise programme, which will increase your metabolic rate, meaning your body will 'burn' fat at a greater pace.

 when you reach the second plateau, try to reduce the fat or oil content in your diet and see if you lose any more weight; it will only be a small drop.

QUITTING SMOKING

Start following this weight loss plan as soon as you quit smoking. It will help control your appetite and reduce your stomach acid. Kadu tea (see page 145) is helpful, and the yogic breathing exercises (see pages 121–3) will help your lungs to function better and eliminate mucus and coughing.

SLOW BUT STEADY

A rapid shedding of weight can be greatly cheering because it appears to be achieving your whole aim, which is to get rid of all your unwanted fat. But a sudden drop is not a healthy sign, as it will probably have been achieved by either depriving yourself of valuable nutrients or following a diet that cannot be sustained.

It may be less exciting to measure your weight loss in tiny increments, but is a much surer, safer way to get lasting results. Weight lost quickly is likely to be followed by weight gained again just as quickly, and a constant yo-yo effect can be as bad for your health as remaining overweight. Your body will not know what to expect next and will start to take precautions against the next 'famine' by laying down fat deposits that will prove even more difficult to shift.

Similarly, if you are battling to lose weight you may think you can never go too far, but dieting and exercise can be an addiction just like chocolate or alcohol. It is not advisable to drop below a BMI of 18. The simple advice is: lose enough weight to look and feel good but never overdo things for the sake of vanity alone.

🍎 After this you should adopt a diet of moderation and follow the advice in Chapter 17 to maintain your new, lower weight.

You may still be above your target weight, but remember that the greater amount of exercise will have increased your muscle bulk and even given you stronger, heavier bones. Rather than using only your weight as a gauge, check your waist measurement periodically: if that reduces even though your weight doesn't, then you are continuing to lose fat while gaining muscle bulk and denser bones – an excellent, positive sign.

There are three elements to this weight loss programme: fasting, control over what you eat and exercise. They work together to:

- reduce appetite
- control sugar and fat intake
- control cravings
- improve discipline and will-power
- create a feel-good factor and the desire to continue
- relax the mind
- exercise the body.

CASE STUDY

In March 2004, the producers of the *Richard & Judy* TV show approached me to treat three patients with chronic illnesses where conventional medicine had failed to provide any answers. One of these was Paul Jackson, whose consultation was filmed for Channel 4.

Paul was in his mid-fifties, weighed 115 kg and suffered from sleep apnoea, back problems, breathlessness and chronic fatigue. I found his neck very stiff, his stomach acid high, signs of candidiasis on the tongue and fluid retention. He used to be a boxer and hits to his head and face had prompted regular neck jerks or whiplash.

I put Paul on my weight loss programme and he received three sessions of neck massage.

Three weeks later he was filmed again. He had lost nearly 8 kg in weight and his face shape had changed. He felt better, his appetite and cravings for sugar had dropped and he was extremely pleased with the way he looked. This was broadcast, and both Richard and Judy praised me live on their show for the brilliant results. That was a pleasant tribute to my work. Paul continued to lose weight after the programme, as he was motivated to follow the plan.

fasting

Set aside one day a week to fast. Consider your lifestyle and choose a day that suits you best. It is quite possible to carry on a day's work if it is not highly physical, but you may prefer to choose a weekend if you have strenuous weekday commitments.

During your fasting day you may have fruit (except citrus or sour fruits), water, fasting tea and vegetable soup. If you prefer you may go on a more restricted fast, of only water with honey and lime.

For more on fasting tea, permissible fruits and how to make the most of your day of abstinence, see Chapter 9.

Follow this fasting programme for four or five months.

what to eat

This diet does not put restrictions on quantity: it only avoids those foods that are known to have ill effects on the body (sugar in excess, coffee, alcohol, canned products, yeast, etc.).

You can eat everything else that is not on the 'avoid' list, so your meals can include meat, eggs, vegetables, rice, pasta, potatoes, fish, many fruits, and non-yeast bread such as soda bread. This makes it an effortless and easy plan to follow as you can live on these things very comfortably without feeling deprived. It is a healthy way of eating and after you have avoided coffee, citrus fruits, alcohol, chillies and so on for several months, you may find that you get bloating, anxiety, headaches or other unwelcome reactions if you reintroduce them into your diet.

Because your basic problem is a matter of eating too much for the amount of energy you expend, it is particularly important that you follow the advice in Chapter 10. This way, you will conquer cravings, avoid over-stimulating your appetite and learn a new appreciation of food. Your stomach will contract.

Following this healthy eating plan will accentuate your body's sensors, so in fact you are only helping your body to keep itself healthy. You are respecting your body and it is doing the same.

Do make sure that you don't cut down on your fluid intake, especially water. Aim to drink at least 1.5 litres a day, but avoid drinking a lot of water while you are eating, as I believe it dilutes the digestive juices. For added interest you can flavour water with a little fruit juice or a drop of vanilla extract. Herbal teas are also a pleasant alternative, and there are many different ones available. One I particularly recommend as part of a weight loss plan is kadu and kariatu tea (see box, opposite).

FOODS YOU SHOULD AVOID

- yeast products: bread made with yeast (including naan, pitta and pizzas), yeast-based spreads and gravy mixes
- citrus fruits, sour fruits, summer berries, rhubarb: see page 104 for a more complete list
- vinegar
- canned foods and ready-prepared food in sachets or bottles (ready-to-mix sauces, ketchup, tomatoes, baked beans, soups)
- coffee
- alcohol
- chocolate, cakes, sweets, sugar (use a little honey to sweeten tea if you wish)
- fried food
- nuts
- butter, cheese
- mushrooms
- curries, chillies and other very spicy dishes
- fizzy water and canned drinks, squashes, bottled juices.

KADU AND KARIATU TEA

These herbs make a bitter tea that is used as a detoxifying agent. They keep candida growth in check (see page 41) and prevent the absorption of excess glucose in the gut, which is good for weight reduction. They reduce sugar cravings and improve bowel movement, and can help to stimulate bile secretion. I have used these herbs for almost two decades and find them effective for a number of common ailments. It was patients who tried them who pointed out their effect on reducing cravings or appetite – this is perhaps due to the bitter taste of the alkaloids they contain, which act as neutralizers on stomach acid.

Soak ⅓ tsp or 2–3 twiglets of each herb overnight in a cup of hot water. In the morning, add a little hot water to potentize the brew, strain off the twigs or powder and drink the water on an empty stomach.

exercise and massage

🍎 A suitable exercise regime will depend on your state of fitness and degree of overweight. Begin at a realistic level, but work out a structured plan that increases by graduated stages, so you can see how your stamina, strength and suppleness are improving: this may be a few minutes more walking each day, so many extra laps of the pool, or additional yoga asanas. Chapter 11 has more advice on this.

🍎 Have a regular neck massage once or twice a week, done by a partner, friend or professional (see pages 133–5) to loosen tight muscles and improve circulation to the subconscious brain.

🍎 Find time to relax. Stress can trigger cravings and bad eating habits, as well as increasing stomach acidity (see page 35). Yoga, massage and just taking time out to listen quietly to music can all help you unwind. Feeling good helps reinforce your determination to reach your goal.

other aids

🍎 A good multivitamin and mineral formulation will help to boost energy levels.

🍎 Chawanprash is an old Indian tonic that contains plant extracts. It provides a natural supplement of vitamins, minerals, and other nutrients (see page 164)

🍎 Gokhru tea (see page 208) will help with fluid retention.

why does this plan work?

Rather than simply prescribing, or proscribing, certain foods, it is the lifestyle changes encompassed in this plan that enable you to lose weight effectively. It is the better eating habits, massages to improve

CASE STUDY

A middle-aged nightclub owner became breathless and nearly choked at a football match as he was trying to climb a flight of stairs — an ambulance was called and he was taken to hospital. He feared a heart attack, but tests proved his heart was not the cause of his trouble. However, he was warned that, at 105 kg, he was grossly overweight. A mutual friend, whom I had helped in the past, sent him to see me.

He confessed that he often craved sugar and did no exercise. I put him on a general weight loss plan, which meant no acidic fruits, coffee, yeast, over-spicy food or alcohol, and gave him weekly neck massages. His weight dropped markedly and in four months he had lost almost 16 kg.

Although that scare at the football match was not due to his heart giving out, his excess weight was certainly a strain on his heart and would have put his life in danger sooner or later if he had not taken steps to lose the weight. He believes the weight loss plan he followed was a lifesaver.

blood flow to the pituitary–hypothalamic area of the brain, reduced hunger pangs and cravings, and an enhanced feel-good factor thanks to relaxation and exercise that cause the weight loss, because making these adjustments allows your body to rectify itself using its own self-regulatory system.

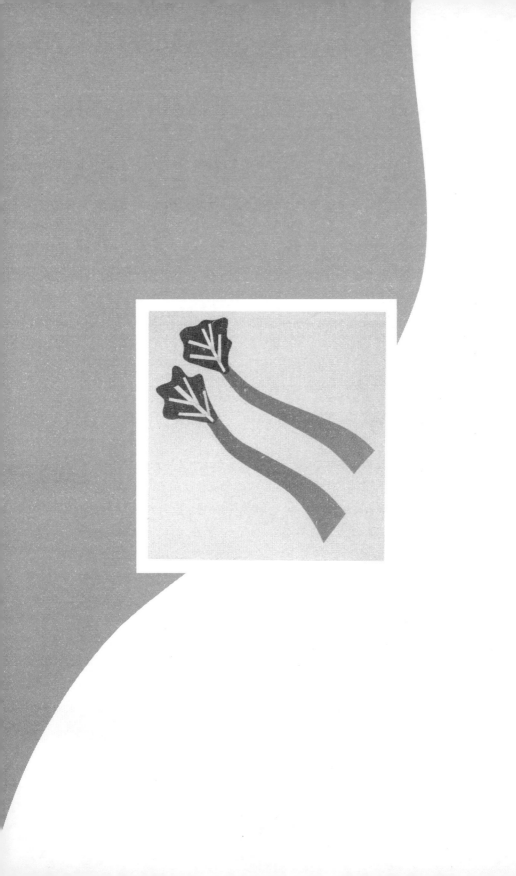

If You Have a Hormonal Imbalance

The number of people in this group is growing and they are accepting this as a part of life. They try all sorts of diets, appetite suppressants and even resort to liposuction and fat-burning electrical stimulators. Often, these do result in some weight loss, but the weight quickly comes back, and with it a growing frustration. You begin to wonder if all the effort and money was worth it. The main winners here are the manufacturers: the powders, the shakes, and the gadgets are all part of a massive weight loss industry with powerful and seductive marketing strategies.

Weight that is predominantly hormonal in origin is the most difficult to shift and so only drastic measures and persistent effort can change things.

Let us look at the problem. The weight you have put on is of three different sorts:

🍎 yellow fat, which your body has stored as an energy reserve that has not been called on

🍎 white fat (cellulite), manufactured to store reserves of the female hormone oesterone (especially but not exclusively in women – see page 27)

🍎 fluid retention, caused by pituitary–hypothalamic, kidney or lymphatic system malfunction.

The yellow fat can be reduced by giving your body less to store (diet control) and burning up the stores by increasing the demand for energy (exercise), but the other contributors to your excess weight will not respond to a simple diet and exercise regime since they have been brought about by biochemical changes in the body. Only methods that reverse such changes will work to shift the weight.

Is it possible to make your body change in this way? In my first-hand experience over many years I have noted that the following all cause people to lose significant weight by biochemical alteration:

🍎 prolonged fasting, for perhaps three weeks or more

🍎 certain extreme diets: zero- or extremely low-fat; high-protein; high-protein, high-fat and zero- or negligible carbohydrate

🍎 extreme worry or stress

🍎 fat-burning drugs

🍎 chronic ailments leading to poor appetite

🍎 chronic diarrhoea causing malabsorption

🍎 high thyroid function or excess doses of thyroxine, increasing the metabolic rate (to the extent of causing palpitations, sweating, diarrhoea and muscle tension).

Now, obviously, most of these are not the route to happy, healthy weight loss, but they do show what the body is capable of. Close analysis of what is influencing the body changes in these circumstances has led me to formulate methods that normalize the hormonal function and/or break down cellulite fat biochemically. Improving hormonal balance will also assist with the loss of yellow fat, as a poorly functioning thyroid leads to a weak metabolism, making it hard to 'burn off' this type of fat too.

Obesity that is due to hormonal problems responds to a long fast (about two to three weeks) under medical supervision or, if this is not possible, to a zero-fat diet. A specific diet plan has to be adhered to for six months, otherwise the root cause of the problem may remain unchanged and you will soon be back where you started. So the programme for combating hormonal weight gain is a tough one and requires a lot of planning, effort, perseverance and determination. It is not easy, but it will work.

Before you begin such a plan, you must keep in mind the following:

🍎 your hormonal balance is a condition over which you have no direct control, as it is part of your body's involuntary system. You are dealing with something quite difficult so you will need patience and tremendous will-power. Use whatever works best for you to help in this struggle of mind over matter, whether it be prayers or meditation or yoga relaxation techniques – remember that trained yogis can even control their body temperature and heart rate

🍎 do not get frustrated if the results do not come that easily, but do persevere

🍎 never for a moment forget that you have a goal before you and you have to achieve it. You will need to learn to discipline yourself, especially when your diet and exercise regime gets interrupted or temptations seem overwhelming.

THE EFFECT OF HRT OR STEROIDS

Chapter 3 explains how one of the side effects of these drugs is a tendency to put on weight, sometimes quite marked. Steroids increase the fat deposits over the body generally and especially on the face. HRT weight gain, on the other hand, causes white fat deposits (cellulite), typically below the belly button, on the buttocks, thighs, arms and below the breasts.

When taking these drugs, keep a close check on your weight right from the beginning; it will be a bit of a fight, but less so than trying to lose a great deal of weight that has built up. For damage control:

- eat slowly
- avoid acid-producing foods (see pages 35 and 104)
- have regular neck massages (see Chapter 12)
- exercise in the gym regularly and/or do yoga exercises daily
- eat your evening meal early.

After the drugs have been stopped, go on a regular weight loss plan such as that described in Chapter 13, with a once-a-week fast.

The best plan to offset the effects of HRT is a zero-fat or very low-fat diet or high-protein, low-starch diet (see pages 155–61 and 162–65).

fasting

By fasting, you are forcing your body to draw on its energy stores in order to keep going, because you are not providing it with food. After using up the reserves of glucose (stored as glycogen in the liver), your body soon begins to consume or 'burn up' yellow fat. It is only after the yellow fat has been consumed that the body will turn to the white fat, cellulite, for sustenance.

When the healing crisis is reached, between the ninth and eleventh day of fasting (see page 99), the body is desperate for energy and breaks down the resistant white fat. It is at this point that fasting becomes particularly effective for overweight with a hormonal cause. During the healing crisis and after, the cellulite deposits become softer and fat disappears from the buttocks, lower abdomen, thighs and so on. The loss in weight and size becomes much more noticeable as up to this point the loss has been predominantly from fluids and yellow fat.

The reason that people with hormonal weight problems find weight loss fasting programmes at health farms or clinics so disappointing and ineffectual in the long term is that most advise fasting for five to seven days. Over this period the healing crisis is never reached and the persistent white fat remains untouched.

The first stage in losing weight, therefore, is a long fast of between 14 and 21 days, if this is possible. It is only by going through the healing crisis that the necessary biochemical changes will be triggered. On pages 98–101 there is a description of the different stages you can expect when fasting.

FASTING SAFELY

I cannot emphasize strongly enough that a fast of this type should only be undertaken under the specialist supervision of a physician experienced in managing long fasts. A strict fast longer than seven days (i.e. without even fruit or soups) should never be attempted without proper facilities and qualified medical care. It should not be attempted at home, even as an outpatient under the guidance of a naturopath or nutritionist. Fasting safely and successfully over a long period requires assessment of mental attitude as well as physical well-being, and only an experienced physician should decide how long a patient should go on fasting or stay on a minimal diet.

A semi-fast can be extended to two weeks at home, but keep a regular check of your BMI (see page 86). Should it drop to 21, you should be monitored closely by a physician with either frequent visits or consultations or in a clinic situation where regular check-ups can be carried out.

At the end of the initial fast, you will be guided to reintroduce foods slowly back into your diet. After this initial period of readjustment, you will need to plan your longer-term eating habits.

If the facilities for a long fast are not available, there are other alternatives which are also effective, but will take longer to show the effects. I advise:

🍎 an initial three-day fast, and then one-day fasting once a week (see Chapter 9).

🍎 a restrictive diet (see below), to be followed for at least six months.

the next move

On the following pages are two diet plans, one in which fat is severely restricted, and one in which starch is very restricted.

Each needs to be followed strictly for six months or, ideally, 12 months. Biochemical changes in the body take time to kick in, so you have to follow the plan and not cheat. You will be tempted, and other people will tempt you, to 'break the diet just once, nothing will happen'. This is just not true. This is not like a calorie-counting diet in which you can make up for a lapse one day with extra restrictions the next. Every time you break the diet you break the biochemical process and have to go back over old ground to reach the same point.

In conjunction with modifying your eating habits, exercise and massages (especially of the neck) are an essential part of the plan (see Chapters 11 and 12). Successful weight loss is about lifestyle changes, not only about food. That is why this plan is different and has greater and more lasting results.

zero- or ultra low-fat diet

In this dietary plan, fat or oil intake is severely restricted but protein and carbohydrate intake can be normal or nearly normal. Restricting your protein and carbohydrate intake at the same time will achieve speedier weight loss, but it is important that you do not do this for more than three months.

A very low-fat diet puts the body under great strain, especially if it is followed for a period longer than three months. As well as energy reserves, the body needs fat to manufacture chemicals essential for day-to-day functioning and a healthy immune system. When little or no fat is forthcoming from dietary sources, the body then breaks into its fat reserves, including cellulite, to synthesize the necessary cholesterol and fatty acids.

GETTING THE BEST FROM THE DIET

This diet works best when you adhere to the basic principles. The first couple of weeks are the hardest; after that you will get used to food without fats and begin to enjoy the new way of eating. As a bonus you will digest food better and have no gas or abdominal discomfort. The weight loss will encourage you: you will feel light and never want to go back to oily or fried food again. Also remember that the diet is a healthy one as it helps to remove deposits of cholesterol or lipids in the arteries. This is good for your heart and blood pressure and can help prevent stroke and circulatory problems. The improved blood flow to the brain, muscles, heart and other tissues is invigorating and makes you feel good.

What to eat

Since the emphasis is on minimal fat intake, you will have to cut out most meats and dairy foods and all fried food.

Avoid:

- red meat and prepared meats such as ham and sausages
- duck and goose
- skin from poultry and fish
- butter, cheese, cream, milk and other dairy products except a modicum of low-fat yoghurts and some low-fat milk for tea or cereals
- any foods prepared in oil or fat, including oil-based salad dressings.

Meal ideas

Breakfast: Bread is usually not a good choice as it really needs accompaniments like butter and spreads. Instead, choose:

- boiled eggs
- cottage cheese with crushed walnuts or cashew nuts
- oatmeal porridge cooked with soya milk
- fresh fruit chosen from the list on pages 104–5.

COPING WITHOUT FAT

Fat-free diets often taste quite bland and leave you feeling not quite satisfied after a meal. About 60 per cent of Indians are vegetarians and know from their long experience of cooking fine vegetarian food that ghee (clarified butter) and oils enrich the flavour of dishes and take a long time to digest, making a meal more satisfying. Many vegetarians rely on cheese for adding a rich smoothness and a feeling of fullness: a vegetarian diet without cheese is digested very quickly and soon leaves you feeling hungry again, and overweight vegetarians often respond quickly to a low-fat diet.

So, fats provide more than just the obvious calories to our diet; they satisfy our senses with their smoothness and richness (of both touch and taste) and leave us with a feeling of fullness. How can we compensate for this on a virtually fat-free diet?

- Thick soups based on pulses and lentils are both filling and pleasingly smooth on the palate
- Avocado gives a good sense of fullness and is satisfyingly creamy. Although it is high in fat, this is of vegetable origin, so permissible in moderation
- Nuts also satisfactorily line the stomach so, well-chewed and again in moderation, nuts can help prevent hunger pangs.

Much of our food derives its flavour from fat, whether intrinsically, added in cooking methods such as frying and roasting, or from accompanying sauces or dressings. Cutting out almost all fat and relying mostly on boiling, steaming and baking as ways of cooking can result in a very bland and unappealing diet unless you enhance the taste as much as possible in other ways. Eastern cooking has the answer to this, as adding herbs and spices enlivens the flavour and also improves digestion. Remember that you have to stay on this diet for six months to achieve optimum results, so it is important that you do not get bored with this cookery style. Do all you can to make the food as tasty as possible without the use of oil or fat or excess sugar.

Low-fat preparations often contain fat substitutes. We do not know how some artificial products used for this purpose may affect our bodies so, like sugar substitutes, they are best avoided.

Lunch and dinner

- lean white meat (skinless chicken or turkey)
- eggs
- lean game
- some offal, such as kidney, calf's liver
- fish (again, no skin) – the fat in oily fish is not a problem, but cooking in oil is
- plenty of vegetables
- a complex carbohydrate: rice, potatoes, pasta or yeast-free bread.

Spicy meat or fish: Marinating your meat or fish before cooking is a marvellous way of adding real flavour to a meal so that you will not miss the fat. Mix up any of the following combinations (and experiment with others) into a paste:

- garlic, onion, ginger, black pepper and salt
- garlic, coriander and green chillies (not too fiery)
- garlic and dill leaves
- fresh tomatoes, onions, garlic, ginger and mustard
- garlic, ginger, paprika powder, turmeric (just a pinch), powdered clove, cinnamon and cardamom
- onion, ginger, a little garlic and saffron stamens.

Make incisions into the meat or fish to allow the flavours to penetrate, and leave to marinate for 30 minutes to an hour before grilling or baking.

SLIMMERS' MASHED POTATO

Cook the potatoes in plenty of water and rinse thoroughly afterwards to reduce the amount of starch. Mash the potatoes with salt and black pepper, and for creaminess you can add a little soya milk or low-fat milk. Stir in herbs or finely chopped spring onions for extra flavour.

LOW SALT

Since meals on a low-fat diet are inclined to be bland, many people find they are using more salt in order to enhance the flavour. It is very easy to exceed the recommended level of salt a day (about the equivalent of 1¼ tsp), and a high salt content in your diet is not a good idea for several health reasons. Among other problems, it may cause fluid retention which, of course, hinders weight loss. Use herbs and spices to bring extra taste to your food, but a moderate amount of potassium-based salt-replacement or 'low sodium salt' is permissible.

These marinades also work well with vegetarian substitutes such as tofu and soya cubes.

Drink herbal teas: liquorice with a little fennel has a sweet taste and makes a refreshing tea.

Flavour-packed lentils with meat: Soak the lentils for two hours. Add to a pan of water with cubed chicken or lean game, garlic, ginger, chopped tomatoes, turmeric powder, paprika and chopped coriander leaves. Bring to the boil and simmer until cooked. Stir thoroughly. This lentil dish can be eaten with rice or as a soup.

Hotch-potch: This makes a simple and filling soup that can be eaten throughout the day. Just put together in one pan chicken or fish, washed basmati rice, potatoes, chopped leeks, carrots and onions (all chopped), garlic, ginger and black pepper, and boil together until everything is thoroughly cooked.

Fat-free stew: In a pan, stew cubes or chicken breast or fish with chopped garlic, ginger, cinnamon sticks, cloves, cardamom pods and

DRY SKIN

One minor side effect of this diet is that your skin may feel dry. Rather than dousing yourself in oil or heavy moisturizer after a bath, which blocks the pores, rub a good massage or body oil (see page 208) all over your skin 10–15 minutes before a shower or bath, and then use a very mild soap when washing. Using oil before bathing moisturizes the skin more effectively and if you do it regularly then your skin feels naturally moisturized.

some whole black peppercorns. When cooked, add a little cornflour to thicken the sauce.

If you do not like a lot of onions and garlic and strong-tasting spices, meals will inevitably be blander, but that does not mean they need be tasteless; indeed, your tastebuds will become attuned to the more subtle tastes of good-quality food unmasked by additional flavourings. Herbs impart a wonderful range of flavours to meat and fish without the bite of spices, so be adventurous with them. Here are a few ideas:

🍎 oven-bake whole fish (wrapped in foil to keep it moist) packed with fresh lemon or orange thyme and a little crushed sea salt and black pepper

🍎 grill fish steaks over stalks and heads of fennel, or chicken over thyme or marjoram

🍎 add a little tea and a variety of herbs (dried or fresh) to the water when steaming diced chicken or turkey

🍎 wrap meat or fish fillets in sorrel leaves before cooking

🍎 make a stuffing from a mixture of herbs, breadcrumbs, salt and pepper, bound together with a little beaten egg. Use this to fill pockets cut in thick cuts of meat or in the centre of thin rolled fillets.

CASE STUDY

Carol, now in her fifties, came to see me about 10 years ago. She weighed 20 stone – a truly obese woman. She had tried every possible diet, had lost weight on occasion but put it right back on when she stopped following the diet. She had pains in her hip joints and knees and was constantly breathless. In her teens she had had several falls from horses and she had started gaining weight since then.

Having diagnosed that her weight problem had a hormonal root, my main role was to motivate her. I told her she could not follow my programme because she did not have the will to do it. She rose to the challenge and immediately made up her mind to prove me wrong – this was the first vital achievement: determination to go through with it.

Since she could not go to a naturopathic centre for a long fast, I counselled her to fast for three days, initially, and then one day a week. She also followed a low-fat diet for six months, initially also restricting her starch intake. She came for neck and back massage twice a month and walked for exercise, as she was too heavy to do any other form of exercise at that stage.

Her weight fell steadily and she had to change her wardrobe several times as her size shrank. After six months Carol had lost 3 stone, and at this stage she plateau'd. I encouraged her to do spot massage with oil and to exercise. She joined a gym and massaged the lower abdomen and sides of the thighs where the main cellulite deposits were. However, she felt too embarrassed to go to the swimming pool as her diminishing figure was so unflattering. She approached her medical insurance company for cosmetic surgery. When they refused I wrote a strong letter pointing out that her weight loss had reduced the risk of hip and knee replacements, heart disease, stroke, diabetes, vascular clots and leg ulcers, among other things. Her effort was saving them money. Someone sat up and took notice, because they paid for her cosmetic surgery – the first time any insurance company had done so.

Carol now looks fantastic and has kept the weight off.

high-protein, low-fat, low-starch diet

This is a slow but steady way of losing weight from hormonal problems. It should not be confused with the popularly marketed high-protein, *high*-fat, *no*-carbohydrate diet (see pages 165–6); this is a practical diet that, with the right motivation, you can adapt (with a once-a-day addition of a complex carbohydrate such as rice or pasta) to stay on long-term.

What to eat

Unlike the near-complete exclusion of fats in the previous diet, a controlled amount of vegetable oils in cooking, such as olive, corn or sunflower, expands the cooking repertoire and makes it simpler to produce tasty meals.

Eat:

🍎 between 250 g and 400 g of protein-rich foods a day. This equates to two chicken thighs or two thick fish steaks

🍎 plenty of green salad ingredients: lettuce, rocket, radish, celery, watercress, spring onions. When these are raw they help to tenderize protein and aid its digestion

🍎 leafy greens and stems, such as asparagus, broccoli and cauliflower

🍎 plenty of fresh fruit from the list on pages 104–5.

The protein and vegetables will give you enough nourishment and

PAPAYA

These beautifully coloured exotic fruit, now widely available, contain papain, an enzyme which is a natural meat tenderizer. Eating papaya in the morning will help you digest protein and unripe papaya can be grated into stews. It also has a mild laxative effect.

ESSENTIAL ROUGHAGE

To compensate for the low amounts of complex carbohydrates, include 'neutral' roughage (i.e. not from fruit or vegetables high in sugars) in your diet from:

- leafy greens
- psyllium husks (1–2 tsp stirred into water and swallowed quickly before they set into a gelatinous mass; drink more water to flush them down)
- bran flakes (without sugar)
- porridge.

Constipation may interfere with your successful weight loss, so sometimes it is worth taking a mild laxative with senna to ease the bowels.

satisfaction. The fruits will give you vitamins and minerals together with simple carbohydrates (fructose), which get metabolized very easily. No one becomes obese with fruits. (Mangoes, bananas and grapes might normally contribute to weight gain, but that is when you eat too much of these together with other carbohydrates. In this dietary plan, the fruits should be a welcome source of necessary nutrients.)

Avoid:

- complex carbohydrates (starches):

    rice

    pasta

    bread

    pulses

    frozen peas

    potatoes, parsnips and other starchy root vegetables

    pumpkins and squashes.
- fats in excess (butter, cheese, cream, fatty meats).

CHAWANPRASH

Chawanprash (see page 208) helps elimination and provides nutrients which one may overlook during this period of restraint. This traditional tonic is full of nutruents from natural sources

Meal ideas:
- grilled chicken breast with stir-fried vegetables
- fish soup made with lots of vegetables; ginger, garlic and cinnamon would be good flavourings
- poultry or lean game (such as pheasant or rabbit) casseroled with a variety of vegetables added towards the end of the cooking time
- Low-starch rice (see box, opposite) would be an acceptable addition from time to time.

Marinades for chicken or fish
All the marinades given on pages 158–9 are suitable here, and you could add a little olive oil for extra flavour. Try also:

- yoghurt, garlic, ginger paste and black pepper
- mustard, garlic, onion, a few drops of lime juice and a teaspoonful of olive oil.

Grind or mix to a paste in a blender. Cut grooves in the skinned meat or fish and rub in the paste well. Leave to marinate for 30 minutes or so before cooking under the grill or in the oven. (Cover with foil first to avoid burning and then uncover to let the marinade dry out a little.)

Although these diets will have a slower effect than a high-protein, no-carbohydrate diet, you will nevertheless experience a slow but steady

---

LOW-STARCH RICE

Wash the rice well first and cook it in plenty of water – about 2.5 to 3 litres of water to 200 g of rice – and boil for 15 minutes. Transfer the rice to a sieve or pasta strainer and rinse thoroughly in boiling water to wash off the excess starch. This rice is almost as tasty as when traditionally cooked but the reduced starch makes it ideal for a weight loss plan.

---

weight loss. Moreover, you will not regain the weight quickly when you graduate back to a regular diet, and there are none of the serious health complications of some other weight loss plans.

about a high-protein, no-carbohydrate diet

There is no doubt that this is a fast and easy way of losing weight, and what people want most is to lose weight without any effort. How is it so effective and what is it doing to your body?

A typical high-protein, no-carbohydrate diet includes bacon, eggs, cheese, steak, sausages, lamb chops, poultry, citrus and berry fruits as well as some salad and stir-fried vegetables (not potatoes). The diet excludes all potatoes, pasta, rice, sugar, pulses, bread, chocolate, cereals, etc. This is not a diet on which you are likely to feel hungry, as proteins and fats are digested slowly, creating a longer-lasting sense of satisfaction after eating, and only those who crave sugar might find it a bit of a challenge. Eating out is not a problem as you can always find meat and vegetables or salads on the menu.

The biochemical change that takes place within the mitochondria, the power stations of the cells, is a complicated one, but basically, with no carbohydrates to convert into glucose for energy, the body is 'tricked' into believing that it has gone into starvation mode. In response it rapidly begins to break down fat, first yellow fat and then cellulite. The fat that is consumed in the diet has no chance of getting stored. Actually, you do not need this dietary fat except that it gives flavour to food and makes the diet an easier and more appealing one to follow.

There is a debate going on about the pros and cons of this diet, but common sense will tell you that this eating pattern cannot be good for you. Unfortunately, it has been marketed as a quick fix for weight problems and there is no doubt about its efficacy: But at what cost? Here are some of the complications that I have noticed:

- a rise in urea, creating kidney problems and gout
- high cholesterol levels from excess fat consumption
- irritability
- bad body odour and bad breath from excessive protein consumption. Our natural body odour increases when too much meat or protein is consumed. And here is a little something to think of: meat-eaters, whether lions and tigers, African tribal hunters or Supermarket Man, will always choose meat from herbivorous rather than carnivorous animals as the flesh of meat-eaters has a very strong smell and is nowhere near as tasty as that of grass-eating animals
- constipation.

This is an ideal diet for those who want to risk health hazards for the sake of losing weight.

don't forget ...

As well as regulating *what* you eat, you must also follow the advice on *how* to eat. Here is a quick checklist:

CASE STUDY

I was called to see the Chief Executive of a major American clothing company, who had been bed-ridden with backache for almost two weeks. On examination I found his kidney area extremely sore to touch, yet he said it was his lower back that bothered him. He could not lie on his back and the pain got unbearable at night so he could not sleep. I asked him about his diet. He said he was on a popular high-protein diet, with which he had lost almost two stone.

It was obvious to me that his kidneys were the cause of his backache. Kidneys are embedded within the lumbar muscles so when they hurt (due to dehydration or malfunction), the muscles in the entire lumbar area hurt and you get very painful stitches. His was not a disc-related backache.

I put this gentleman on a two-day semi-fast, allowing him only fruit and soup and 2 litres of water a day. I gave him gentle massages and simple yoga exercises. After the first day of fasting his pain disappeared like magic. It was the diet he had been following – high protein, high fat and no carbohydrate – that had caused his kidneys to ache and the whole area to be so painful.

🍎 eat slowly

🍎 avoid over-stimulating your appetite (see Chapter 10)

🍎 avoid eating late in the evening (ideally, have your evening meal by 7 p.m.)

🍎 avoid the 'five evils' (yeast and fungus, alcohol, coffee, citric or sour foods, excess sugar) as far as possible: these either interfere with your digestive ability or consist of calories without nutritive value, or both. See Chapter 10.

eating out

Eating out while on a diet is never going to be as easy as preparing your own food, and you may find it simpler not to socialize for the first couple of weeks while you get used to your new diet and feel the first benefits of it.

🍎 *On restaurant menus,* be guided by what complies with your diet restrictions and don't be sidelined into all your old favourites. Look for an interesting salad (if you are cutting out fat completely, make sure you get it without dressing) or a consommé or clear soup as a starter. Among the main courses you can usually find poached or steamed fish; choose this with steamed rice or vegetables, or just leafy vegetables if you are on low carbohydrates. Even if all the options seem to come with rich sauces, the kitchen will probably be willing to provide a plain grilled or steamed dish if you explain what you cannot eat. For dessert, fresh fruit (see pages 104–5) is a good choice – without cream, of course. And pass on the cheeses.

🍎 *If you go out to a party* where a buffet meal is served, then choose carefully, opting for green salads, cold cuts of poultry and so on. Plain rice is fine on a zero-fat diet, as are beansprouts, sweetcorn and raw vegetables cut for dips (just avoid the dips). If you find chicken or fish in a rich sauce, you could avoid this, or at least try to leave as much sauce behind on your plate as possible.

🍎 *When eating at somebody else's house,* it is tempting to break your diet rather than not eat what everybody else is eating. This is where you need to call on your will-power and determination. Talk to your host or hostess beforehand to let them know your dietary restrictions. Eat what you can and be strong about avoiding what you cannot eat. Sometimes it is worth eating something to suit your dietary plan before you go for dinner, so that hunger pangs do not weaken your will. If it is appropriate, offer to bring something suitable along that they can serve you. Alternatively, invite people round to your home and enjoy the company while keeping control over what you eat.

🍎 ***Get in the habit*** of taking suitable food with you to work or when you travel, so that you do not have to rely on finding something appropriate 'on the hoof'.

Once you have reached your target weight, you have to be very careful about the diet and exercise programme. In four to six months you get used to eating in a certain way. See Chapter 17 for how to maintain your optimum weight.

The low-fat option can be a permanent one. There is no harm in eating like that. You can lose all the fat you want. Since this diet incorporates carbohydrates there is no danger at all. When you have lost the desired inches or weight, stay on the low-fat diet and increase the carbohydrate content (porridge, fruits, pasta, ordinary rice without the starch being washed off). The weight will stabilize and you will continue to feel and look great.

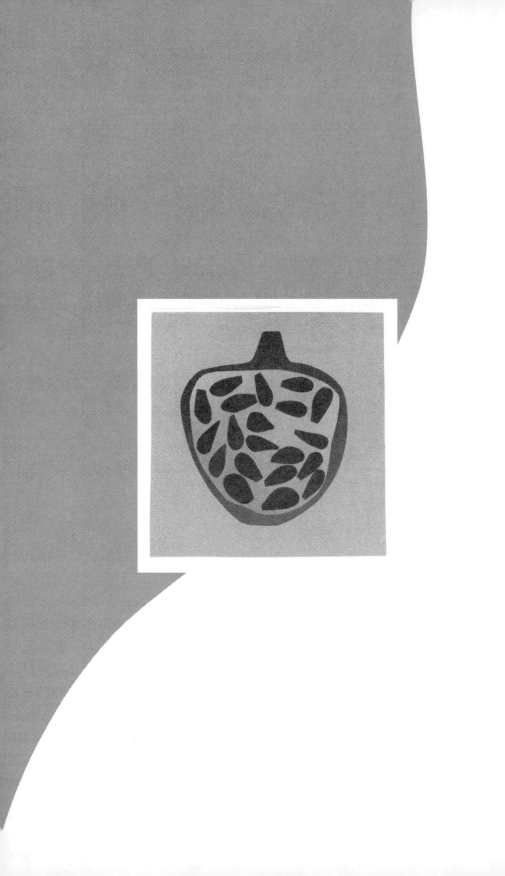

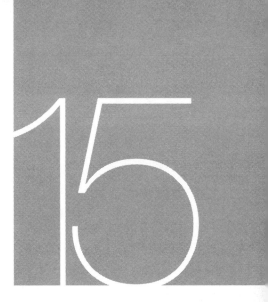

If Your Overweight is Familial or Genetic

If over half the members of your family are overweight, then you will need to sit down together and draw up a strategy. Approaching excess weight as a problem for the whole household is much more effective than each individual trying to follow their own path.

As explained in Chapter 1, the familial link can be influential in many ways. From the Self-assessment (see Chapter 8), you may have deduced whether the excess weight is due mainly to diet and lack of exercise, or whether the main problem is hormonal. Depending on your answer, you should follow the weight loss plan described in either Chapter 13 or 14. There are several further steps you can take to help offset the contribution that family traits or genes make.

family meals

In general, we come to think of what we grow up with as the norm, but it is very helpful to try to look at some aspects of family life more objectively.

amounts of food

Following the advice in Chapters 10 and 13 will help retrain your stomach to eat less, but for a family who has always eaten large amounts and is used to seeing a plate piled high, making adjustments is going to take time and effort.

how much is a portion?

How do you know if your meals consist of normal or supersize portions? Apart from cheese and other dairy foods, which you will have cut out, or right back on, as part of your weight loss plan, it is usually with meat and starchy foods that many families are over-generous. It may help to consider the following:

🍎 a portion of meat is about 75 g – a piece about the size of a pack of playing cards

🍎 a portion of rice (cooked) is 2 rounded tablespoons, or 3 rounded tablespoons of pasta or noodles.

Learn what an appropriate portion looks like on the plate – it may help to weigh or measure the main items of each meal for a few days. Always

MORE ON CARBOHYDRATES

Just as we are encouraged to eat at least five portions of vegetables and fruit every day, we need a variety of starchy carbohydrates as well, about six portions in all (but not all the same).

1 portion =

3 tbsp breakfast cereal

half a bagel or pitta bread

3 crackers or rice cakes

1 medium potato

2 oatcakes

1 thin slice of bread

If you were to have a large bowlful of cereal for breakfast, a couple of rounds of sandwiches at lunchtime and three or four potatoes or a heaped plate of rice for supper, you could easily consume 10 or more portions.

serve by counting spoonfuls and looking at the amount on your plate before adding more, rather than filling the plate.

For everyone to reduce their servings is not only a healthy move, but it is a considerate gesture to those in the family who are striving to lose weight.

the store cupboard

Convenience plays a great part in what we eat. If a packet of crisps or the ingredients for a cheese sandwich come to hand more readily than fruit or a potato to bake, then, typically, that is what we'll go for.

Agree on a list of foods not to buy, but for each Don't Buy, substitute a Do Buy – your weight loss plan may founder early on if you constantly

BITTERNESS: THE APPETITE SUPPRESSOR

Most people do not like bitter tastes and are put off food instantly even when they are hungry. In India, various bitter-tasting vegetables are used to help suppress appetite, and some are even recommended for control of diabetes. The bitter taste in these vegetables and herbs come from alkaloids, which neutralize acid in the stomach, so suppressing the appetite.

feel hungry or deprived. Take account of all the family's special downfalls, especially if you are prone to snacking – if you know they are there you will be tempted to eat them.

Instead of:	*Have:*
🍎 sweets	vegetables that can be eaten raw (such as carrots, celery, mangetout)
🍎 cakes and sweet biscuits	low-fat, low-sugar biscuits
🍎 cheese	fruit that you all (or at least some of you) like – easy, 'pop-in-the-mouth' fruit such as grapes, cherries and physalis are useful ever-ready snacks
🍎 sweet or fizzy drinks	whole fruit juices (preferably non-citrus) and flavoured mineral waters (try out different ones as they vary a lot in taste)
🍎 creamy desserts	low-fat yoghurts

Add to this list any other foods that you commonly have in the house but which hinder rather than help weight loss – see the 'Avoid' list on page 144 of Chapter 13 and also the information in Chapter 10.

cook's tips

Whoever does the family cooking has extra responsibility. A series of small changes can, together, make a surprising difference to the family diet. Try the following:

- whenever possible, bake, steam or poach rather than fry
- use an unsaturated oil such as olive or sunflower rather than butter or lard
- if a meal needs a creamy sauce, use low-fat crème fraîche or yoghurt rather than full cream
- calculate beforehand how much food you actually need for the meal – many cooks, especially when catering for a growing family, have got into the habit of always 'doing a little extra, just in case'. Avoid this trap of encouraging overeating
- don't automatically put out sauces and 'extras' on the table. If the sugar, the ketchup, the mayonnaise, the butter are not within arm's reach, it will help everyone who is trying to lose weight. (Better to ban them from the house altogether!)

EXPAND YOUR RANGE, NOT YOUR WAISTLINE

Instead of automatically buying the familiar, plan to try at least one different thing each week. It might be a new type of fruit (the range of exotic fruits in supermarkets is growing all the time) or a new dish – when did you last have peppered chicken in a yoghurt sauce or home-made fish cakes? TV cookery programmes and their spin-off books, magazines and even free recipe cards in supermarkets are all heavily leaning towards healthier eating and provide a wealth of inspiration.

family life

In some families each person goes their own separate way, but others are more close-knit and do things together. This can be a boon or a burden when attempting to follow a new lifestyle plan. Sitting and watching TV all evening and sharing beers and crisps may be convivial but it can make breaking the mould all the harder.

Harness the enjoyment you get from each other's company by doing something more active – perhaps going swimming one evening a week, or signing up for classes in tennis or yoga (or something more unusual such as fencing or kendo). Or organize family rambles or bike rides. These are all good forms of exercise to do alone, but doing them as a family brings extra support and encouragement. It will also help prevent the younger members of the family from succumbing to familial-induced obesity.

worries about obese children

Excess weight can be a problem at any age, but in children the familial links are often a particularly strong influence.

Overweight children are much in the news these days, and North America is not the only place where childhood obesity is a major social concern. In Britain the National Study of Health and Growth (1974–1994) reported that obesity in children has increased substantially since the mid-1980s. While genes and hormones account for some of the problem, much more is the result of overeating and poor nutrition.

Responsibility lies both with parents and schools, and anyone else who is *in loco parentis*. The providers of food to children should ensure that the children in their care eat healthily, both in terms of quality and quantity. In addition to introducing a healthy eating regime at home, what can you do to help?

🍎 Ensure that food is the focus of attention at mealtimes: don't let TV or computer games be a distraction or your child will not learn to recognize the 'I'm full' signs their body sends them.

🍎 Train your children not to gobble down their food: as we have seen, eating slowly is an invaluable habit.

🍎 Raise the issue of diet at school. This is a matter of increasing concern at all levels, and schools are much more susceptible to parental pressure and campaigning than they were even a few years ago.

🍎 Regular massage of the neck and shoulders helps to keep appetite under control and is of particular help to children for whom birth trauma

CASE STUDY

Through the shock of her own son's weight increase a friend of mine in Boston became involved in the problems of obesity in teenage children in the neighbourhood. She noticed that they ate large meals, snacked on high-calorie food and drank colas all day long. These children grew lazy and did little but watch TV in their spare time. Many of them were exempted from games because they were too large.

She was concerned about these children growing up to be obese men and women obsessed with food. She discussed the matter with nutritionists and began giving talks and lectures to motivate the children. That had little or no effect.

Then she came upon a different approach: with the agreement of the local schools she employed a nutritionist for them, to provide tasty but low-calorie meals. She also set up a fund that would provide free meals where required. The results were heartening: the children began to lose weight. Plans are now being drawn up to involve children in games and sport, with the expectation that this will be successful over the next few years.

Setting up charities and funds to help schools provide healthier and leaner food for children is one way of getting down to the grass roots and tackling obesity in society.

or subsequent injury to the neck may be causing problems of blood circulation through the vertebral arteries (see Chapters 6 and 12).

 Involve your children in healthy eating research. You might ask them to look up things online. What they discover for themselves is much more likely to impress them than what they are told.

Suitable foods and meal ideas for children of different ages, from newborns to teenagers, are covered in more detail in my *Nutrition Bible*.

If overweight is a common family trait, whether through nature or nurture, then the same tendency is likely to show up in the next generation. Even if your children are young and skinny now, they have a greater than average chance of being saddled with the same weight problems later on, quite possibly when they reach puberty. Being fore-warned of this is a great advantage and gives you the chance to instil healthy eating habits and an active lifestyle that will swing the balance in your child's favour.

puppy fat

The hormonal upsurge of puberty is often accompanied by increased weight, coming at just the wrong time, when a half-grown child is faced with so many other pressures and changes to come to terms with. At times like this, all four main types of weight gain, including psycho-logical, can come into force at once.

Good eating and lifestyle habits learned earlier will stand a burgeon-ing pubescent in good stead now, but as a parent you may find it helpful to read the next chapter as well – comfort eating or surreptitious binge-ing do not have to reach the stage of a psychological problem before they become a threat to weight. An unbiased third party, such as a trained nutritionist, may also be an asset, to avoid food and eating becoming a 'home hang up'.

as you grow older

In old age, we are all inclined to gravitate towards thinness or fatness. If you have watched your own parents, grandparents or other relations of previous generations get stouter and stouter it is probable that you will be prone to do the same. Habits become increasingly difficult to break the longer we have them, and as you go through your sixties, seventies and eighties you may find you are inclined to keep to the same regimes and menus that you have had all your adult life. However, in many other ways your life and your body will have changed greatly and once you pass 60 it makes sense to review what, when and how much you eat.

Your digestive system will not have maintained the miraculous elasticity and robustness of a 20-year-old, so pamper it a bit.

🍎 Have a good breakfast and make lunch your main meal of the day, with just a light supper.

🍎 Avoid too much rich, spicy food.

🍎 Cut down on saturated fats, such as cream and cheese.

🍎 If you are only catering for yourself, pre-packaged ready-made meals may seem like a dream come true (and some are), but check labels carefully, as acids and emulsifiers can upset the system, and many are more loaded with sugars and fats than you might realize.

Balancing the amount you eat with the amount of energy you expend is as important now as at any age. How much you exercise may depend on how much you have done in the past, the state of your joints and general suppleness, but even mild, regular daily movement will decrease the amount that will get stored as fat. Walking is good all-round exercise, and many places run yoga, tai chi, Medau and similar sessions specifically for older people.

Neck and shoulder massages a couple of times a week are also a great help, both to ease stiffness and to help with the cravings for sugar or food in general.

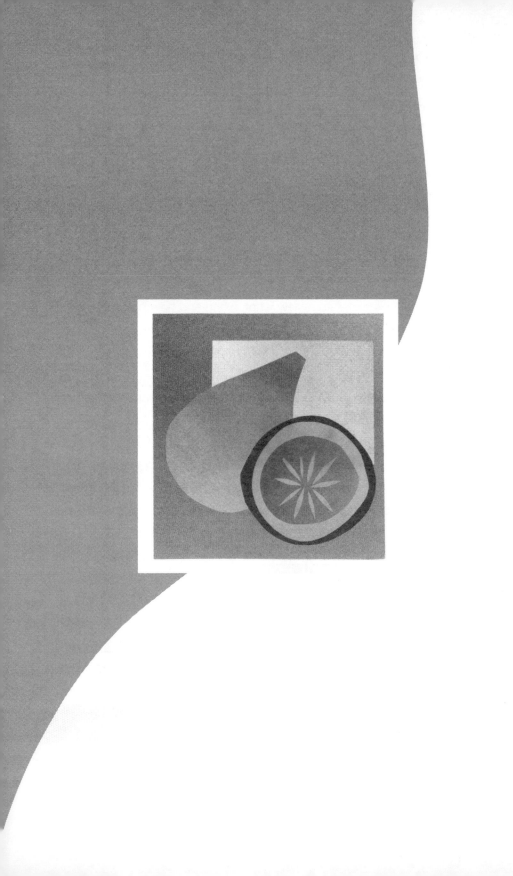

If You Have Psychologically Related Weight Problems

Most of us have turned to food or drink as a comforter at one time or another, and in almost every office you will hear somebody say something like: 'I just can't function until I've had that first hit of caffeine/my morning doughnut.' Food can certainly affect our minds, as we have seen in Chapter 7, but for some, eating becomes an automatic response to stress or unhappiness and the two become inextricably associated. This may manifest itself by the actual act of eating, putting

CHRONIC FATIGUE SYNDROME

CFS has been given such names as 'yuppie flu' and, since many of the symptoms are psychological, has frequently been categorized as a psychiatric disorder and treated with antidepressants. I believe that CFS is a multifactorial condition (see page 11) with psychological implications. Since CFS saps you of all energy (sometimes even making movement of any sort difficult), it can result in a weight increase from lack of exercise, which can bring on mild or severe depression. Depression from the nature of the illness may also trigger over-eating.

food in the mouth, or of turning time and again to a particular food (typically something nutritionally unhelpful, such as chocolate).

Extreme stress, damaging low self-esteem, a distorted view of one's own body or deep psychological disturbances are primarily a matter for psychological treatment, but when they become bound up in the mind with food, obesity becomes part of the problem. Eating more food than your body requires is not going to leave you physically unscathed. Gaining large amounts of weight contributes to the distress, depression or guilt, and so perpetuates an ever more frustrating and dangerous spiral. Keeping weight under control can be part of the solution.

damage control

Your first approach should be damage control. You may not be able to conquer your desire to eat, but the *quality* of what you eat will have an effect. That simply means eating things that will satisfy your hunger and fulfil your need to eat while having as little effect as possible on your weight.

Give yourself two simple dietary rules:

 at mealtimes eat protein and salad or boiled/steamed vegetables at all other times stick to non-citrus fruits, plain yoghurt and dried fruits.

With this eating pattern at least some control can be exercised while you work through the psychological problems.

the value of protein

Eating protein for breakfast, lunch and dinner will provide a greater sense of satisfaction from eating and, because it is digested more slowly, keep the stomach fuller for longer. This will relieve any pressure to eat from hunger pangs and make it easier to control the number of times you want to eat.

Strict vegetarians and vegans find it particularly difficult to reach that feeling of satisfaction, as most of their diet is so easily digestible. Eating too much cheese is not a good solution. To achieve that necessary sensation of a full stomach, the following are helpful alternatives:

EAT AS MUCH AS YOU LIKE OF...

 grilled fish or chicken with steamed vegetables

 cold chicken breast with a mixed salad (include carrots, cucumber, cherry tomatoes and lettuce) with a yoghurt or olive oil dressing

 boiled egg on a bed of salad with fresh vegetables and boiled corn

 chinese-style chicken or seafood soup with oriental vegetables (baby corn, bean sprouts, bamboo shoots, etc.)

 lentil soup (very filling) and cold chicken breast or grilled fish/chicken

 cottage cheese with crushed walnut and a vegetable soup

 salad with prawns and avocado.

QUICK-TIME MEALS

Keep in stock plenty of:

- chickpeas, kidney beans and other pulses (available canned in water)
- sardines, salmon and other fish canned in oil or brine.

Use these as the basis for almost instant, filling meals: try any number of different combinations using rice, tomatoes, spring onions, herbs and spices, with any of the foods listed in the box on page 183.

- avocado
- soaked almonds
- bean sprouts
- exotic fruits that are slow to digest: lychees, fresh coconut, jackfruit, durian, custard apple.

taking it slowly

As explained elsewhere, eating slowly gives you an important control over your food intake. Psychologically induced eating patterns force you to eat fast. Controlling that urge is very therapeutic. You will feel satisfied and eat less.

Put a timer beside your plate and make each meal last 20 minutes. Chew each mouthful well; savour the food, don't bolt it. Put your knife and fork down between each mouthful.

Before beginning each meal, spend a minute of silence in front of it. You could either make this a moment of prayer or spend it in contemplation of what is on your plate. This draws your attention to the food and diverts your mind from whatever is concerning you at other times. Divorcing the two is very good practice.

Don't drink copious amounts of water straight after a meal. Wait

CASE STUDY

Jane was three stone overweight. She had an abusive father and was teased at school for being slightly chubby. She lost confidence in herself. Whenever she was stressed she used to eat. After a few years it became a regular feature and by the time she came to see me at the age of 30 she had tried every possible diet that she could, but could not stay on them for long. Her mind worked out every meal ahead of time. She would feel very hungry long before mealtimes and eat a lot. She snacked when tired or stressed.

As I have done with other patients, I challenged her and said she did not have the will-power to help herself. She was upset and wanted to prove me wrong, which is just what I wanted her to do.

Within days her personality changed. She took up my yoga and relaxation regimes, had neck massages and made great progress. She fasted one day a week on fruit and water, schooled herself into eating slowly, and avoided heavy dinners and all the foods she was recommended to steer clear of. She also took up swimming regularly.

Jane's food binges stopped and her weight just dropped off: in five months she had lost her excess three stone. Colleagues at work and her friends began to praise her looks. That increased her confidence and she was able to overcome her psychological difficulties.

for 30–45 minutes to allow your gastric juices to work at full strength on the food.

massage

From my experience of dealing with psychological weight gain, I have found neck massage very useful. These are the benefits I have noticed:

🍎 neck massage improves the blood flow to the limbic system where many of the brain's emotional centres are located. Weekly therapeutic massage using my technique has a calming effect, reduces anxiety and depression and helps control mood swings. In this feel-good state the triggers to binge are less

🍎 neck massage also improves the blood flow to the pituitary–hypothalamic area, reducing food cravings and controlling appetite. Bingeing on food becomes less aggressive

🍎 for bulimics, who binge and then vomit, the urge to make themselves sick comes from a psychological guilt association and a physical feeling of nausea. In interviewing bulimics, I found that almost 90 per cent had had some accident involving the neck (whiplash, head injuries, etc.) one to five years preceding the problem. Working on the neck helps to reduce the nausea after eating and reduces the urgency to vomit. (See Chapter 12.)

relaxation

The mind has phenomenal power to heal itself. Just as the physical body heals cuts, wounds, burns, bruises, and so on, emotional problems can also be healed by laying down the ideal conditions.

To keep its innate healing power in good shape, the mind needs sleep, proper nutrition and mental exercise.

Good and restful sleep can do a great deal to calm the emotions. There is a lot of argument about the number of hours we should sleep. Doctors used to prescribe eight hours of sleep but now they say seven hours is enough. My opinion is that, although there is a minimum requirement, it is the quality of sleep that matters most. An afternoon siesta or catnap can help to break the day into two halves and regenerate the energy, both mental and physical, to perform better. If the brain 'ticks away' all night then it will use up its reserve energy and get exhausted. The daytime performance gets affected. It is more likely to get stressed.

THE MIND IS WHAT YOU MAKE OF IT

Electrical impulses and neurotransmitters, which chemically transmit messages from one nerve cell to another, control the functions of the brain. Just as these chemicals can be stimulated with emotions, they can also be regulated with controlled thoughts.

Swami Ram Lakhan, the yoga master who features in my Lifestyle DVD, is 90 years old but looks 20 years younger. He eats once a day, sleeps for just three hours every night and wears no woollens or warm clothes in winter. With his mind he can slow down his pulse rate to 40 beats per minute, hold his breath for up to 30 minutes and can make his hands cold or hot at will.

There is no doubt that relaxation and meditation helps to calm and still the mind. Start with a simple relaxation method that will teach you to breathe correctly, concentrate and divert your mind to different parts of the body in a sequence. You may then progress to meditation. Regular practice will harness your wild thoughts and bring changes in your behaviour. This will give you the ultimate relaxation that you look for.

It takes patience and perseverance to overcome eating problems, whether they are bingeing, obsessive compulsive eating or bulimic behaviour, but mastering a relaxation or meditation technique will help you be able to say, enough is enough.

seeking help

When your mind is in turmoil you cannot always focus, make the right decision and have the will-power or motivation to face things on your own. Unfortunately, people are so busy with their own lives that they have very little time for others. But professionals – psychiatrists, counsellors and psychotherapists – are there to help. Seeing these

CASE STUDY

As the daughter of performing parents, Zara led a peripatetic life and was often on her own in the evenings. Eating staved off the boredom and by the time she was nine years old she was already overweight. In her early twenties she became a vegetarian and an obsessive exerciser, but after a back injury she had to stop exercising and her weight slowly crept up again. When she met a man she loved, she was motivated to lose weight again, taking up exercise and trying a variety of diets. However, in her mid-forties she suffered a bereavement and her relationship broke up, which brought on major depression. She became virtually bedridden with ME (a severe form of chronic fatigue syndrome) and gained over 12 kg in a year. She also had an underactive thyroid but was not taking any medication. Things worsened as she approached the menopause. By her early fifties she weighed just over 100 kg and her cholesterol level was high, even though she was still a vegetarian and tried to avoid too much fat.

When Zara saw the *Richard & Judy* show on TV in 2004 (see page 142), she bought my *Nutrition Bible* and came to see me. I put her on a very low-fat diet, demonstrated the neck massage that would improve her hormonal balance and asked her to go for walks, as she could not do much exercise due to the chronic fatigue. I told her there would be no point in her coming to see me again if she couldn't stay on the diet.

She was disturbed that I underestimated her will-power. She followed my diet plan and her partner gave her a neck massage once a week. She came to see me after 12 weeks and smiled as she walked in: she had lost 12 kg. She begged to be allowed some oil into her food as she craved flavour, but I told her to continue with the same programme. I saw her again 10 weeks later, when she had been following this strict regime for five months. She had lost more than another 6 kg and was thrilled with her reduced measurements: 15 cm lost from the buttocks, 10 cm from the hips and eight cm from the bust. Her fatigue was still preventing her from walking much, but I said she might use oil for an occasional stir-fry as long as she increased her walking, so that she didn't start putting on any weight.

Being overweight can often be due to more than one clear-cut cause and for Zara a habit of snacking begun in childhood, irregular exercise, hormonal problems and comfort eating had all contributed to her weight problems.

specialists, especially in conjunction with a weight loss plan integrating diet, exercise, and massage and relaxation techniques, will be of great assistance in your motivation and journey back to health.

What you have is an illness as real as any physical one. Do not deny that you have it and do not let embarrassment prevent you discussing an eating disorder with friends or relations. They can help you in many ways. Ask them to encourage you to:

- practise a relaxation technique
- do the yoga programme
- stay on a weight loss plan
- avoid proscribed foods
- keep up the physical exercise.

Such support and encouragement is invaluable, especially when things seem bleak or your will fails you.

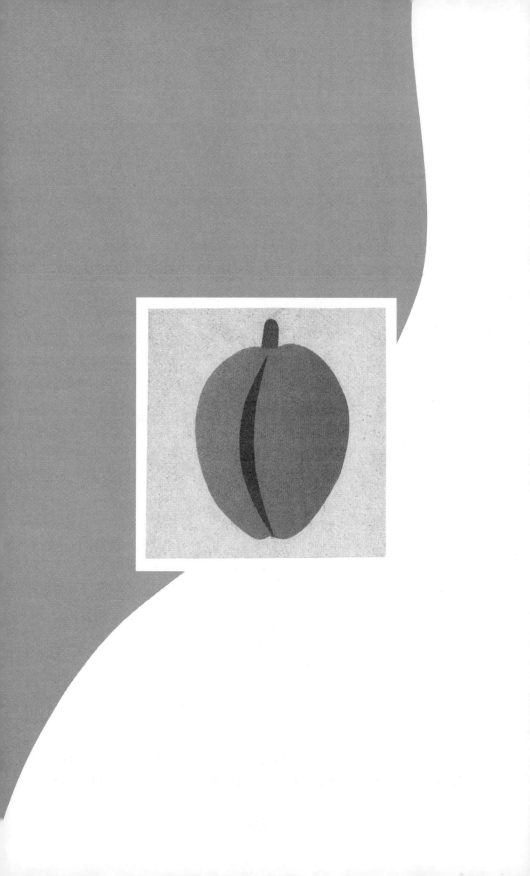

17

Maintaining Your Optimum Weight

Time after time, I hear tales of frustration from people who, having worked hard to lose weight, find it inexorably creeping back up again. They are understandably depressed and find it difficult to recover the will to start all over again. It is like building a sandcastle on the beach only to have a huge wave come and wash it all away.

Keeping your weight at a desirable level is even more important than losing it in the first place, and experience of my own weight loss plans shows that weight gain afterwards is very slow or non-existent. Here are the reasons why.

 The plans involve a whole change in lifestyle, not simply a short-term dietary modification – massage and yoga, alongside diet, are an integral part of my plans. Because of this you will notice a general improvement in health and a sense of well-being that encourages you to continue.

🍎 With a retraction of the stomach walls and a new-found awareness of your body's messages, you reach a state of feeling satisfied much earlier, and so you are inclined to eat no more than you need.

KEEPING UP THE GOOD WORK

Once you have reached your optimum weight, eating in moderation and regular exercise is often enough to stay there, since your body and mind are now naturally attuned to an appropriate diet and level of eating. Make the following part of your regular, lifelong regime:

🍎 weekly massage

🍎 once a week fast, or occasional three-day fasts

🍎 daily exercise.

Your success will also help you maintain the will-power you need. And you can use simple methods of self-regulation:

🍎 if you overeat at one meal, compensate by eating only very light food for the next two meals

🍎 weekly fasts are an excellent way of keeping your eating habits and your weight in check. Fasting helps you to connect spiritually with your inner self

🍎 eat according to your body type (see Chapter 8).

Weigh and measure yourself regularly, so that you spot any weight increase early on. Measuring your waist (also chest for men, and hips and thighs for women) is useful because weight alone does not differentiate between the comparative contributions of fat, muscle and bone. As you age, bones lose density and account for less of your overall weight, and so even a small increase in weight in an older person can indicate a greater increase in fat.

🍎 Neck massages help control the appetite centre, which means that food cravings drop.

🍎 Appetite is further regulated by control over excess stomach acid.

🍎 Yoga, relaxation and motivation enhance the feel-good factor, encouraging sensible eating so that bingeing, cravings or addiction to food lose their hold.

There is no quick fix to reaching and maintaining a sensible weight. You need to allow time to retrain your body and your mind, and I recommend staying on your chosen dietary regime for a minimum of four months, and longer if you can.

hormonal weight gain

Overweight or obesity that is caused primarily by a hormonal imbalance is not only the most difficult to reduce, but also means a lifelong regime to keep it under control. You will always need to monitor your weight very closely.

Having followed a strict diet for perhaps six months, your body will have got used to a quite different way of eating. Now you will need to consider how to go on from here.

The low-starch diet is not one that can be adhered to forever, so make the addition of one portion a day of a complex carbohydrate such as rice, pasta or potatoes. A typical day's food might consist of:

breakfast

🍎 eggs *or* cottage cheese with almonds (soaked for 24 hours)

🍎 non-citrus fruits *or* a high fibre cereal such as porridge, muesli or branflakes

🍎 tea

lunch
- fish and vegetables
- soup

dinner
- chicken or fish (lean meat twice a month) with vegetables with herbs/spices
- potatoes or pasta with rice

(you can interchange lunch with dinner)

The low-fat diet can be a permanent one if you increase the carbo-hydrate content: porridge, bulgur wheat, noodles, couscous, potatoes, pasta, ordinary rice without the starch being washed off

breakfast
- eggs (poached or boiled)
- porridge
- fruits (non citrus)

lunch
- steamed/grilled fish or chicken breast (continue to follow fat-free flavouring ideas from the low-fat diet, pages 155–60)
- steamed vegetables

dinner
- same or variation on lunch with a carbohydrate (boiled or steamed)

Adopting either of these regimes, together with the lifestyle changes you have already undertaken – regular massages, exercise and relaxation, will keep your weight stable and enable you to continue looking and feeling great.

HELPING WITH IMBALANCES

There are certain natural products that can help with an imbalance of hormones. Seaweed contains iodine, which is necessary for the proper functioning of the thyroid, so I recommend sea kelp tablets for hypothyroidism.

For problems related to oestrogen imbalances, as might occur during the menopause, I recommend Shatavari, which can be taken in capsule form. This helps regulate hot flushes and irritability as well as weight increase.

stumbling blocks

Those who have lost weight through my plans find it quite effortless and easy, and some have made it their regular eating pattern for life, helped by the entire lifestyle programme incorporating exercise and massage.

However, it would be unfair to paint a fairytale picture and say that, once you have reached this stage, you will never face problems or temptations again. Your long-term plan from now on should reflect what you recognize are your own difficulties, depending on your general circumstances and temperament.

Unwillingness to exercise

This is a very common problem. Although following gym routines or doing exercises by yourself at home can indeed be effective, many people find them very boring. The few yoga *asanas* described in Chapter 11 barely touch on a form of exercise that is highly rewarding both physically and mentally, and there is no end to the challenges that yoga can present.

However, your new lighter weight will have opened up all sorts of novel possibilities that you may not have considered – you may need to adjust to the idea that you are no longer somebody who can't play badminton, go ice-skating or learn to tap dance!

🍎 Think laterally: if doing lengths of the pool is uninspiring, find out if there is a local scuba-diving club. Jazzercise may not be your cup of tea, but have you thought about belly-dancing?

🍎 Joining a club or society adds a new dimension to exercise, as it provides welcome encouragement and motivation: in addition to team sports like football or volleyball, there are organizations devoted to almost any form of exercise you can think of, from hiking to orienteering.

🍎 Martial arts, despite the rather militant-sounding label, encompass a number of very different disciplines, ranging from the graceful, almost yoga-like tai chi to energetic ju-jitsu.

🍎 Walking, swimming or cycling to raise funds for a charity is a great motivator.

🍎 Incorporate as much movement as you can into everyday life: walk rather than take a lift or escalator; walk your young children to school rather than drive them; consider walking or cycling instead of always driving or taking a bus or train.

Comfort eating

Old habits die hard, and it is when our emotions are stirred up, whether they stem from nervous stress or unhappiness, that we are most likely to seek reassurance from familiar comforts – just like an older child might revert to thumb-sucking.

Regular or frequent lapses of this sort particularly need guarding against if a hormonal imbalance was the original cause of your over-weight, as a one-day fast or semi-fast may not compensate sufficiently.

A two-pronged attack may help here:

🍎 The first is to identify what is causing you to turn to food for comfort: is it an ongoing problem such as constant work pressures or a failing marriage, or periodic stresses such as exams looming or unwelcome visits from in-laws? If it is not so easily identifiable, you may need to keep a record of events, noting feelings alongside what you eat before you spot the trigger or triggers. Solving the stresses and strains of life is far beyond the scope of this book, but recognizing what is endangering all the good you have achieved is a first step, and will fuel your determination to resolve the problem, either alone or with the help of friends or professionals.

The second is to find some other, innocuous 'comfort blanket' that can stand in for food while the problem is sorted out. This will be a very personal choice, since it needs to have all the right comforting associations to do the job. Here are some comforters that have provided the answers for some people:

- immersion in a warm, scented bath
- phoning a friend
- a long walk
- playing a musical instrument
- hugging a childhood teddy
- an absorbing craft such as painting or model-making
- replaying a favourite heart-warming film or piece of music.

Inability to resist temptation and a love of food

Overcoming this is definitely a case of mind over matter. Again, it is an extra problem if you have had to cope with hormonal weight gain, as simply compensating by eating very lightly or fasting for a day may not, after a while, be enough to maintain your weight.

If you know that there are certain 'forbidden' foods that are your downfall, you will always need to take special care to avoid them being put in your way – this may mean banning them from the house, avoiding particular shops or aisles in the supermarket or making an announcement on the office email: whatever it takes. There are many delicious and nutritious options that, with a little imagination, can replace your old favourites. Make sure these healthy alternatives are close at hand.

If you generally love food and cooking as part of the enjoyment of entertaining and socializing (a typical characteristic of phlegmatics; see below), you may have had to curtail this aspect of your life while on the strictest part of your weight loss plan. Restricting your diet will have increased your awareness of how different foods affect you, both alone and in combination, and made you look anew at the properties of different foods. Turn this to your advantage.

Rather than relying on your old recipes and menus, learn even more about healthy eating, and carry this knowledge through to providing imaginative meals that do not rely on a lot of fats and heavy, rich sauces or hard-to-digest mixtures of ingredients. You will start to look and feel so much better that you will begin automatically to look for lighter ways of preparing delicious meals without feeling that you are depriving yourself of anything.

Family pressures

This can be a constant battle and, as the various scenarios in Chapter 15 suggest, maintaining a healthy weight is a lot easier with the backing and participation of the whole family. If you have been the only one with the weight problem, your family may have been very supportive for months, but may have been counting the days until 'we get back to normal'.

Family life is constantly one of give and take, of compromises, so once you have reached, or nearly reached, your target weight, sit down with your family again and review the next stage. They may have thought that your very restrictive diet would go on forever, or that, once you achieved sufficient weight loss, the days of chips and chocolate cakes would reign once more. It will be helpful to explain what you need to do to maintain your new, slimmer self.

CONVINCING OTHERS

One of the trickiest problems in maintaining a healthy eating programme is other people. It can be very tough to stick by your guns when faced with: 'Come on, it's not going to make any difference to your diet to have a little of this delicious dessert/just a glass of wine/you've got to try some of this.' You don't want to fall out with friends, and sometimes you feel it would give offence to say 'no'. You may even feel embarrassed, or be laughed at.

Ironically, diabetics, people recovering from a heart attack, or anyone who has a condition that requires a specific diet, receive understanding and sympathy, but in many people's minds 'just being overweight' doesn't fall into this category. Attitudes are changing, but society in general is still not as conscious of healthy eating as it should be – that is why the weight issue is such a major problem in health care. People will not take their weight seriously and often they will not let others do so. Yet, take courage from the fact that taking action now may mean you avoid the life-threatening diseases and conditions that obesity can bring. There is much truth in the old saying: *Prevention is better than cure.*

On your side, you may find that, having conquered cravings for sweet things or a habit of snacking, you no longer find it an unbearable temptation to have in the house things that you can't eat.

following your body type

In Chapter 8 there is a guide to body types, and an explanation of the differing influences of constitution and temperament. While few people are constantly and consistently a single type, you should find that you have an inclination or dominance of one type – although even this is not immutable, and can change with age and circumstances.

Adopting a dietary regime that suits your body type is especially useful if you have a tendency to regain weight quickly. This way, you give your body the nourishment that suits it best and, should you divert from the norm every now and then, following a regime most applicable to your innate self will make it easier for your body to rectify itself.

Melancholics and cholerics are seldom troubled by overweight, so you are most likely to have identified yourself as a phlegmatic, or possibly a sanguine type.

phlegmatic type: Of all the types, phlegmatics have to take the most care over what they eat. As you probably know to your cost, you find it very easy to put on weight and difficult to keep it off. Once you have succeeded in losing weight you will need to be particularly alert to the dangers of putting it all back on again.

The weight loss plan you have followed will have done more than simply reduce your food intake; it will have introduced your body to a whole new approach to food and to life. It is this, far more than any avoidance of specific foods, that will enable you to maintain your new, healthy weight.

🍎 Exercise regularly. Exercise not only keeps weight in check, it creates a feel-good factor that is a huge boost to morale.

🍎 Fast once a week. Fasting helps to build will-power and will be an ally in what may be a lifelong struggle against weight gain.

🍎 Follow the low-fat diet plan as often as you can.

🍎 Keep your motivation strong. At times this may be the most difficult thing. Chapter 16 may be helpful in keeping in perspective any tendency to bingeing or turning to food when you feel down or unhappy.

Avoid citrus fruits, very spicy food, sugars, excess alcohol, excess salt and fats.

sanguine type: since sanguine people are by nature active and can usually eat well without adverse consequences, there are two main guidelines you need to bear in mind:

🍎 you need to be careful about adjusting your food intake to your level of activity

🍎 you should not overstrain your system just because you aren't getting any adverse effects or signs.

An active life builds muscles, which require protein, but it is preferable that this mostly comes from lower-fat sources such as chicken and fish rather than copious amounts of red meat. While you get plenty of exercise, fat in your diet will be 'burned off' or metabolized well, but if your level of activity drops (as it probably will as you get older) this can be a cause of an increase in weight, as well as health problems, so it is better not to get into the habit of relying on fats for energy.

Your digestive system, and particularly the liver, has to work hard to process the results of your hearty eating and a little cosseting will be a great help. Follow the guidance in this book to eat slowly, wait half an hour or so after eating before taking in fluids in any quantity, and avoid eating late in the evening. A rest after lunch and a walk after dinner will also aid digestion.

Do a fruit fast (rather than a full fast) at least once a month, to give your digestive system a respite. The fruit will provide the energy you need in an active day.

A high tolerance to alcohol means you do not get early warning signs or ill-effects, but the strain on the liver and other organs is just as great.

Eat plenty of calming foods, such as cucumber, melon, fresh mint, spinach, pumpkin, courgettes, squash, etc. Drink peppermint or chamomile tea.

Avoid an excess of stimulating foods, such as coffee, salt, game and red meat; and appetite stimulants that will encourage over-eating, such as citrus fruit, highly spiced food, white wine, champagne and brandy (see also page 37).

A LAST WORD ...

Here are some thoughts that might help you avoid the trap of ever getting fat again.

🍎 LOOK at what you are eating. The colours, the presentation and the nature of food should give you a pleasant feeling.

🍎 SMELL your food. The aroma and the distinct smells should give you more pleasure.

🍎 JUDGE your food. Is what you are eating healthy for you or will it give you trouble later?

🍎 PAUSE for a minute before you eat. Give thanks for your food and put aside worries so that you can concentrate on your food.

🍎 TASTE by eating slowly and focusing on the various flavours. Each type of food has its own distinct flavour.

🍎 ENJOY your food. Food gives you pleasure when eaten slowly and in moderation. It gives you pain when eaten fast and in excess.

🍎 ESTABLISH a healthy relationship with your food. You are what you eat.

🍎 LEARN to cook. It is highly enjoyable and creative, and gives you greater understanding of what you put in your body. He or she who puts food on the family table should command great respect and power.

🍎 ENCOURAGE within the family a culture of eating most meals at home, where we have direct control over our food. Everyone can participate in shopping, cooking and washing up, and help build a family bond.

And finally:

🍎 STOP eating when you feel that another mouthful will make you full.

🍎 EXERCISE when you feel lazy and tired.

A PERSONAL TESTIMONY

At the start, I found Dr Ali's diet rather tough going! For three days, no potatoes, rice or pasta, no bread, no sugars, no citrus fruit, no this, no that – as far as I was concerned, the Doc's prescription consisted only of vegetables and water, and a banana in the morning. Little wonder my intestines got angry. By the fourth day, I felt as though I was carrying sextuplets in my stomach. I certainly couldn't move faster than one mph and began arriving at my own dining room at lunchtime, when I was aiming for breakfast.

From Hong Kong I telephoned the Doc, who had decamped to Dubai, to tell him of my woes, but he wasn't particularly impressed or sympathetic. Instead, he said I should persevere and predicted that from my fifth day, I would start to feel better: I did, and lost nine kg within a month! His plan had worked, but what a struggle it had been at the beginning. But then all diets are a struggle and we know how Sisyphus must have felt.

The trouble is the enormous temptation of food, and we need to find mental strength with which to build up our resistance. The Doc helps with this by giving his massage (which is described in Chapter 12). When I had my first one with him, I had been expecting a soothing and relaxing experience – but it turned out to be rather more vigorous than I had expected, and this took a bit of getting used to! However, as time went by I began to feel stronger, both physically and mentally, and now I regularly go back to the Doc for more. He smiles and laughs all the time and we joke a lot, which in itself is therapeutic.

But you should be warned! Every time you lapse in your diet, you automatically go back to the Doc, because he is magnetic. And so once you embark on this book you will be hooked, as I have been for 15 years – but I have scarcely noticed the years go by. I owe so much to Dr Ali and will be for ever in his debt.

David Tang,
Hong Kong

Epilogue

In the prosperous parts of the world, food has never been more varied, more abundant or cheaper, but this welter of choice has made us lazy and unquestioning about it. We may be shocked by stories of children who have no idea that milk comes from cows, but we have all distanced ourselves from the source of our food, so that where it comes from, how it reaches us, and the different seasons have come to mean less than they should. We listen to what food advertisers tell us but not what our bodies tell us. We are watching a generation of children become obese through ignorance and an inability to withstand the barrage of advertising and merchandising.

In the USA, obesity in the population has increased by 30 per cent in the past decade and, as the figures I quoted at the beginning of the book make clear, the picture elsewhere is hardly more encouraging. Obesity has become a major problem for everyone, fat or not, because excess weight carries with it more than just too much fat. Heart disease, high blood pressure, diabetes and many other health problems are linked to weight gain and are often complicated by it. The strain on the body, from heart to back to knee joints, becomes other people's concerns when it leads to extended health care and hospitalization. Weight problems can bring about, or be brought about by, depression, alcoholism and family break-ups, adding to society's ills.

There is a growing will to change. In certain cultures fat has traditionally been seen as a sign of good health and prosperity, but changing times, awareness of obesity-related diseases, and education means that, worldwide, people are becoming more conscious of their weight. But a conflict continues. While it could not be said to be their prime aim, industries as wide ranging as clothing, furniture and chain restaurants all benefit from an overweight population. Even the slimming industry has benefited from people's inability to lose weight – if they were serious, they would have spent more time motivating people to find a permanent solution rather than a quick fix. We are sucked under a spell from which it is difficult to break free.

So, although obesity has tremendous implications on society and its well-being, the responsibility is going to have to rest at the personal level. We must learn to look after ourselves: to eat sensibly, exercise regularly, and release the stress from our bodies with massage and relaxation techniques. I have tried to explain as best I can how my weight loss plan works, and why. I sincerely hope that both individuals and healthcare workers can learn and benefit from it.

Dr Ali's Treatments

To arrange a consultation please contact:
The Integrated Medical Centre
43 New Cavendish Street
London W1G 9TH
Tel: 020 7224 5111   Fax: 020 7317 1600
Email: info@integratedmed.co.uk
Website: www.integratedmed.co.uk

To order any products that may be mentioned in the book or that are listed overleaf please contact:
Integrated Health Products
43 New Cavendish street
London W1G 9TH
Tel: 020 7224 5141   Fax: 020 7224 3087
Email: shop@integratedmed.co.uk
Dr Ali's website: www.drali.com

PRODUCTS

Dr Ali's Lifestyle Programme – DVD

Dr Ali's Weight Loss – DVD

Relaxation with Dr Ali – CD

Bio-Chawanprash

Dr Ali's Fasting Tea

Dr Ali's Gokhru Tea

Dr Ali's Relaxation Tea

Kadu Tea

Kariatu Tea

Dr Ali's Lifestyle Massage Oil

Dr Ali's Cellulite Oil

Dr Ali's Stomach Formula tablets

BioLiv capsules

Shatavari capsules

Sea Kelp tablets

Index

ACKNOWLEDGEMENTS

I am deeply grateful to my friends Ronnie and Jonathan Newhouse, Wendy and Frank Chapman, Gaynor and Johann Rupert, Alfred Bradley, Leo Stroll, Baldev, Sat and dozens of others who gave me moral support to carry out my creative work.

I sincerely thank Caroline Ball for making sense of my late night writings, Carey Smith for her support, Ed Victor for working on my behalf and, finally, Paul Loades and Sophia Opel at the IMC for providing the logistic support to make this book possible.